Clinicians' Guides to Radionuclide Hybrid Imaging

PET/CT

Series editors:

Jamshed B. Bomanji
London, UK

Gopinath Gnanasegaran
London, UK

Stefano Fanti
Bologna, Italy

Homer A. Macapinlac
Houston, Texas, USA

More information about this series at http://www.springer.com/series/13803

Teresa A. Szyszko

Editor

PET/CT in Oesophageal and Gastric Cancer

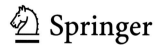 Springer

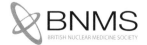

Foreword

Clear and concise clinical indications for PET/CT in the management of the oncology patient are presented in this series of 15 separate Booklets.

The impact on better staging, tailored management and specific treatment of the patient with cancer has been achieved with the advent of this multimodality imaging technology. Early and accurate diagnosis will always pay, and clear information can be gathered with PET/CT on treatment responses. Prognostic information is gathered and can forward guide additional therapeutic options.

It is a fortunate coincidence that PET/CT was able to derive great benefit from radionuclide-labelled probes, which deliver good and often excellent target to non-target signals. Whilst labelled glucose remains the cornerstone for the clinical benefit achieved, a number of recent probes are definitely adding benefit. PET/CT is hence an evolving technology, extending its applications and indications. Significant advances in the instrumentation and data processing available have also contributed to this technology, which delivers high throughput and a wealth of data, with good patient tolerance and indeed patient and public acceptance. As an example, the role of PET/CT in the evaluation of cardiac disease is also covered, with emphasis on labelled rubidium and labelled glucose studies.

The novel probes of labelled choline, labelled peptides, such as DOTATATE, and, most recently, labelled PSMA (prostate-specific membrane antigen) have gained rapid clinical utility and acceptance, as significant PET/CT tools for the management of neuroendocrine disease and prostate cancer patients, notwithstanding all the advances achieved with other imaging modalities, such as MRI. Hence a chapter reviewing novel PET tracers forms part of this series.

The oncological community has recognised the value of PET/CT and has delivered advanced diagnostic criteria for some of the most important indications for PET/CT. This includes the recent Deauville criteria for the classification of PET/CT patients with lymphoma – similar criteria are expected to develop for other malignancies, such as head and neck cancer, melanoma and pelvic malignancies. For completion, a separate section covers the role of PET/CT in radiotherapy planning, discussing the indications for planning biological tumour volumes in relevant cancers.

These Booklets offer simple, rapid and concise guidelines on the utility of PET/CT in a range of oncological indications. They also deliver a rapid aide memoire on the merits and appropriate indications for PET/CT in oncology.

London, UK   Peter J. Ell, FMedSci, DR HC, AΩA

Preface

Hybrid Imaging with PET/CT and SPECT/CT combines best of function and structure to provide accurate localisation, characterisation and diagnosis. There is extensive literature and evidence to support PET/CT, which has made significant impact in oncological imaging and management of patients with cancer. The evidence in favour of SPECT/CT especially in orthopaedic indications is evolving and increasing.

The Clinicians' Guides to Radionuclide Hybrid Imaging pocketbook series is specifically aimed at our referring clinicians, nuclear medicine/radiology doctors, radiographers/technologists and nurses who are routinely working in nuclear medicine and participate in Multi-Disciplinary Meetings. This series is the joint work of many friends and professionals from different nations who share a common dream and vision towards promoting and supporting nuclear medicine as a useful and important imaging speciality.

We want to thank all those people who have contributed to this work as advisors, authors and reviewers, without whom the book would not have been possible. We want to thank our members from the BNMS (British Nuclear Medicine Society, UK) for their encouragement and support, and we are extremely grateful to Dr Brian Nielly, Charlotte Weston, the BNMS Education Committee and the BNMS council members for their enthusiasm and trust.

Finally, we wish to extend particular gratitude to the industry for their continuous support towards education and training

London, UK

Gopinath Gnanasegaran
Jamshed B. Bomanji

Acknowledgements

The series co-ordinators and editors would like to express sincere gratitude to the members of the British Nuclear Medicine Society, patients, teachers, colleagues, students, the industry and the BNMS education committee members for their continued support and inspiration:

Andy Bradley
Brent Drake
Francis Sundram
James Ballinger
Parthiban Arumugam
Rizwan Syed
Sai Han
Vineet Prakash

Contents

Contributors

Kanhaiyalal Agrawal Department of Nuclear Medicine and PET/CT, North City Hospital, Kolkata, India

James Ballinger Division of Imaging Sciences, King's College London, London, UK

Jamshed B. Bomanji Department of Nuclear Medicine, University College London Hospitals NHS Foundation Trust, London, UK

Andy Bradley Nuclear Medicine Centre, Manchester Royal Infirmary, Manchester, UK

Alexis Corrigan Department of Nuclear Medicine and Radiology, Maidstone and Tunbridge Wells NHS Trust, Tunbridge Wells, UK

John Dickson Department of Nuclear Medicine, University College London Hospitals NHS Foundation Trust, London, UK

Gopinath Gnanasegaran Department of Nuclear Medicine, Royal Free London NHS Foundation Trust, London, UK

Ayshea Hameeduddin Radiology Nuclear Medicine, Barts Health NHS Trust, London, UK

Kathryn Hawkesford Department of Medical Oncology, Barts Health NHS Trust, London, UK

Shahriar Islam Department of Radiology, The Royal Marsden NHS Trust, London, UK

Shaunak Navalkissoor Department of Nuclear Medicine, Royal Free London NHS Foundation Trust, London, UK

Anna Paschali Division of Imaging Sciences and Biomedical Engineering, St Thomas' Hospital, Kings College London, London, UK

David Propper Barts Cancer Institute, Queen Mary University of London, London, UK

Angela M. Riddell Department of Radiology/Biomedical Research Centre, The Royal Marsden NHS Trust, London, UK   ·

Evangelia Skoura Institute of Nuclear Medicine, UCLH, London, UK

Teresa A. Szyszko King's College and Guy's and St Thomas' PET Centre, Division of Imaging Sciences and Biomedical Engineering, Kings College London, St Thomas' Hospital, London, UK

Deborah Tout Biomedical Technology Services, Gold Coast University Hospital, Southport, QLD, Australia

Thomas Wagner Department of Nuclear Medicine, Royal Free London NHS Foundation Trust, London, UK

Nilu Wijesuriya Cellular Pathology, Barts Health NHS Trust, London, UK

Introduction and Epidemiology

1

Shahriar Islam and Angela M. Riddell

Contents

1.1 Epidemiology

Oesophageal cancer is the third most common gastrointestinal malignancy worldwide. Over the last 40 years, the UK has seen a rise in prevalence and it is now the 13th most common cancer in adults [1]. It has an incidence of 8,300 new cases each year demonstrating a 2:1 preference for males to females. It is reported that 80 % of new cases are diagnosed in patients over 60 years of age [1]. The

S. Islam (✉)
Department of Radiology, The Royal Marsden NHS Trust, London, UK
e-mail: shahriar.islam@rmh.nhs.uk

A.M. Riddell
Department of Radiology/Biomedical Research Centre, The Royal Marsden NHS Trust, London, UK

© Springer International Publishing Switzerland 2016
T.A. Szyszko (ed.), *PET/CT in Oesophageal and Gastric Cancer*, Clinicians' Guides to Radionuclide Hybrid Imaging, DOI 10.1007/978-3-319-29240-3_1

distribution of tumour subtype varies according to ethnicity with adenocarcinoma favouring Caucasians and squamous cell carcinomas favouring Asian, South American and African populations [2]. Despite advances in multimodality treatment, oesophageal cancer is still devastatingly aggressive with over 65 % of new cases incurable at time of presentation. The disease maintains a 5-year survival of just 15–20 % [3].

There has been a concomitant increase in adenocarcinoma of the gastric cardia, which now accounts for 95 % of all gastric cancers, with the remaining 5 % consisting of a mixture of squamous cell cancers, lymphoma, gastrointestinal stromal tumours and neuroendocrine tumours. Because of the similar gender preference and the affected peak-age group of patients, it has been suggested that adenocarcinomas of the oesophagus and gastric cardia are similar in aetiology [4]. Despite an increase in gastric cardia tumours, the overall incidence of gastric cancer is reducing as a consequence of active health policies to eradicate *Helicobacter pylori* (*H. pylori*) infection.

One of the most established causes of oesophageal and gastro-oesophageal junctional cancers is chronic gastro-oesophageal reflux disease (GORD). Barrett's oesophagus is a recognised premalignant condition involving replacement of normal stratified squamous epithelium within the lower oesophagus with columnar epithelium in response to chronic gastro-oesophageal reflux [4].

Obesity is another recognised risk factor as it predisposes to hiatus hernia and thus acid reflux. The risk of developing a malignancy is 3–6 times greater amongst overweight individuals [5]. Linbald et al. have reported a 67 % increase in the risk of developing oesophageal adenocarcinoma in patients with a BMI >25 [6]. The 'Million Women' study confirmed that 50 % of oesophageal adenocarcinoma cases in postmenopausal women were attributed to obesity [7].

The aetiology of squamous cell carcinoma differs to that of adenocarcinoma of the oesophagus in that it is largely related to poor lifestyle habits, including smoking tobacco, drinking alcohol and a poor diet [8].

1.2   Clinical Presentation/Signs and Symptoms

The main presenting symptom for oesophageal cancer is dysphagia. Unfortunately the symptom frequently presents at a late stage, when the lumen is narrowed to 50–75 % of its normal calibre. By this stage more than 50 % of patients have locally advanced disease [9]. Other symptoms are non-specific and again may go unreported for some time. These include dyspepsia, chest pain, hoarse voice, persistent cough and weight loss.

1.3   Diagnosis

Diagnosis of oesophageal and gastric cancer is made by endoscopy and biopsy. There is a 10 % 'failure to diagnose' rate with patients requiring a second endoscopy [10]. The diagnostic yield to detect high-risk premalignant lesions in Barrett's oesophagus is 100 % when a minimum of six biopsies are taken. Proton-pump inhibitors should be stopped prior to endoscopy as they may heal malignant ulcers and mask their appearances to the endoscopist [4, 11, 12].

1.4 Staging Investigations

The principal imaging modalities for staging are endoscopic ultrasound (EUS), multidetector CT (MDCT) and PET/CT.

1.4.1 Endoscopic Ultrasound

Endoscopic ultrasound (EUS) offers the most accurate method for local staging and is used in patients with localised oesophageal and GOJ tumours who are being considered for radical therapy. It is able to depict the layers of the oesophageal and gastric wall and thus determine the depth of tumour spread through the submucosal layers, allowing identification of patients suitable for local therapy as opposed to surgical resection [13]. The technique also enables fine needle aspiration cytology (FNAC) samples to be taken from local lymph nodes, improving the accuracy of nodal staging [14, 15]

1.4.2 Multidetector CT

MDCT of the chest, abdomen and pelvis is routinely performed as the initial staging investigation. The use of multiplanar reformats in conjunction with axial images has been shown to be particularly useful in accurately distinguishing between T3 and T4 diseases due to the ability to evaluate tumour invasion into surrounding structures [16, 17]. Its primary use however is for detection of metastases. It has a reported 88 % sensitivity and 99 % specificity for detecting liver metastases [18].

1.4.3 PET/CT

PET/CT is now routinely used to refine staging in patients who are considered potentially curable on conventional (MDCT) imaging. It has been shown to detect occult metastases in around 16 % of patients [19]. Recently it has also been reported to be of use in assessing response to neoadjuvant therapy [20].

1.4.4 Other

Laparoscopy is used to assess for peritoneal disease. Direct visualisation of the peritoneal surface can identify 2–3 mm nodules of disease, undetectable on all cross-sectional imaging modalities. It may also detect occult surface deposits on the liver. Its use is advocated in all potentially operable gastric cancer patients and oesophageal patients who have disease extending below the diaphragm.

Currently MRI is reserved for problem-solving, for example, in the characterisation of indeterminate liver lesions [4].

1.5 Staging Classification

The gold standard method for staging utilises a tumour-node metastasis (TNM) classification as defined by the American Joint Committee on Cancer (AJCC) [21]. Cancers of the GOJ and those within the proximal 5 cm of the stomach are staged as oesophageal cancers. Cancers that occur more distally within the stomach are staged as true gastric carcinomas. Specific TNM groups are then classified according to particular cancer stages. These stages provide prognostic information for individual patients. Tables 1.1 and 1.2 give details of the oesophageal staging, and Tables 1.3 and 1.4 below provide detail of the classification for gastric carcinomas.

Table 1.1 AJCC oesophageal cancer TNM staging (7th edition)

Primary tumour (T)	
Tx	Primary tumour cannot be assessed
T0	No evidence of primary tumour
Tis	High-grade dysplasia
T1	Tumour invasion of lamina propria, muscularis mucosae or submucosa
T1a	Tumour invades the lamina propria
T1b	Tumour invades the submucosa
T2	Tumour invades the muscularis propria
T3	Tumour invades the adventitia
T4	Tumour invades adjacent structures
T4a	Resectable tumours involving the pleura, pericardium and diaphragm
T4b	Unresectable tumour involving adjacent structures, e.g. the aorta, vertebral body and trachea
Nodal disease (N)	
Nx	Regional lymph nodes cannot be assessed
N0	No regional lymph node metastasis
N1	Metastases in 1–2 regional lymph nodes
N2	Metastases in 3–6 regional lymph nodes
N3	Metastases in >7 regional lymph nodes
Distant metastasis (M)	
M0	No distant metastasis
M1	Distant metastasis (common sites include the liver and lung)
Histological differentiation grade (G)	
Gx	The grade cannot be assessed
G1	The cells are well differentiated
G2	The cells are moderately differentiated
G3	The cells are poorly differentiated
G4	The cells are undifferentiated

Table 1.2 AJCC prognostic groupings for adenocarcinoma and squamous cell carcinoma

	Adenorcarcinoma				Squamous cell carcinoma				
Stage	T	N	M	Grade	T	N	M	Grade	Location
0	Is	0	0	1	Is	0	0	1	Any
1a	1	0	0	1–2	1	0	0	1	Any
1b	1	0	0	3	1	0	0	2–3	Any
	2	0	0	1–2	2–3	0	0	1	Lower
2a	2	0	0	3	2–3	0	0	1	Upper, middle
					2–3	0	0	2–3	Lower
2b	3	0	0	Any	2–3	0	0	2–3	Upper, middle
	1–2	1	0	Any	1–2	1	0	Any	Any
3a	1–2	2	0	Any	1–2	2	0	Any	Any
	3	1	0	Any	3	1	0	Any	Any
	4a	0	0	Any	4a	0	0	Any	Any
3b	3	2	0	Any		2	0	Any	Any
3c	4a	1–2	0	Any		1–2	0	Any	Any
	4b	Any	0	Any		Any	0	Any	Any
	Any	3	0	Any		3	0	Any	Any
4	Any	Any	1	Any		Any	1	Any	Any

Cancer locations defined as the upper thoracic 20–25 cm from incisors, middle thoracic 25–30 cm from incisors and lower thoracic 30–40 cm from incisors

Table 1.3 AJCC TNM classification of gastric cancer (7th edition)

Primary tumour (T)

Tx	Primary tumour cannot be assessed
T0	No evidence of primary tumour
Tis	Carcinoma in situ: intraepithelial tumour without invasion of the lamina propria
T1	Tumour invasion of the lamina propria, muscularis mucosae or submucosa
T1a	Tumour invades the lamina propria or muscularis mucosae
T1b	Tumour invades the submucosa
T2	Tumour invades the muscularis propria
T3	Tumour penetrates subserosal connective tissue without invasion of the visceral peritoneum or adjacent structures
T4	Tumour invades the serosa (visceral peritoneum) or adjacent structures
T4a	Tumour invades the serosa (visceral peritoneum)
T4b	Tumour invades adjacent structures

Regional lymph nodes (N)

Nx	Regional lymph nodes cannot be assessed
N0	No regional lymph node metastasis
N1	Metastases in 1–2 regional lymph nodes
N2	Metastases in 3–6 regional lymph nodes
N3	Metastases in >7 regional lymph nodes
N3a	Metastases in 7–15 regional lymph nodes
N3b	Metastases in >16 regional lymph nodes

Distant metastasis (M)

M0	No distant metastasis
M1	Distant metastasis (common sites include the liver and lung)

(Continued)

Table 1.3 (Continued)

Histological differentiation grade (G)

Gx	The grade cannot be assessed
G1	The cells are well differentiated
G2	The cells are moderately differentiated
G3	The cells are poorly differentiated
G4	The cells are undifferentiated

Table 1.4 Prognostic groupings for gastric cancer

Stage 0	Tis	N0	M0
Stage 1a	T1	N0	M0
Stage 1b	T2	N0	M0
	T1	N1	M0
Stage 2a	T3	N0	M0
	T2	N1	M0
	T1	N2	M0
Stage 2b	T4a	N0	M0
	T3	N1	M0
	T2	N2	M0
	T1	N3	M0
Stage 3a	T4a	N1	M0
	T3	N2	M0
	T2	N3	M0
Stage 3b	T4b	N0	M0
	T4b	N1	M0
	T4a	N2	M0
	T3	N3	
Stage 3c	T4b	N2	M0
	T4b	N3	M0
	T4a	N3	M0
Stage 4	Any T	Any N	M1

Key Points

- Oesophageal cancer is the third most common gastrointestinal malignancy worldwide.
- Distribution of oesophageal tumour subtype varies according to ethnicity.
- Oesophageal cancer maintains a 5-year survival of just 15–20 %.
- Over 65 % of new cases of oesophageal cancer are incurable at time of presentation.
- Adenocarcinoma of the gastric cardia accounts for 95 % of all gastric cancers.
- Adenocarcinomas of the oesophagus and gastric cardia are similar in aetiology.

- One of the most established causes of oesophageal and gastro-oesophageal junctional cancers is chronic gastro-oesophageal reflux disease (GORD).
- The main presenting symptom for oesophageal cancer is dysphagia.
- Diagnosis of oesophageal and gastric cancer is made by endoscopy and biopsy.
- The principal imaging modalities for staging are endoscopic ultrasound (EUS), multidetector CT (MDCT) and PET/CT.

References

1. Oesophageal Cancer Incidence. URL: http://www.cancerresearchuk.org/cancer-info/cancer-stats/types/oesophagus/incidence/uk-oesophageal-cancer-incidence-statistics. 11 June 2014.
2. Farin K, Wong-Ho C, Christian A, Sanford D. Environmental causes of esophageal cancer. Gastroenterol Clin North Am. 2009;38(1):27–vii.
3. Pennathur A, Gibson MK, Jobe BA, Luketich JD. Oesophageal carcinoma. Lancet. 2013;381:400–12.
4. Allum WH, et al. Guidelines for the management of oesophageal and gastric cancer. Gut. 2011;60(11):1449–72.
5. Cheng KK, Sharp L, McKinney PA, et al. A case control study of oesophageal adenocarcinoma in women: a preventable disease. Br J Cancer. 2000;83:127e32.
6. Lindblad M, Rodriguez LA, Lagergren J. Body mass, tobacco and alcohol and risk of oesophageal, gastric cardia and gastric non-cardia adenocarcinoma among men and women in a nested case control study. Cancer Causes Control. 2005;16:285e94.
7. Reeves GK, Pirie K, Beral V, et al. Cancer incidence and mortality in relation to body mass index in the Million Women Study: a cohort study. BMJ. 2007;335:1134.
8. Zhang HZ, Jin GF, Shen HB. Epidemiologic differences in esophageal cancer between Asian and Western populations. Chin J Cancer. 2012;31(6):281–6. doi:10.5732/cjc.011.10390. PMC3777490.
9. Koshy M, Esiashvili N, et al. Multiple management modalities in esophageal cancer: epidemiology, presentation and progression, work-up and surgical approaches. Oncologist. 2004;9(2):137–46.
10. Yalamarthi S, Witherspoon P, McCole D, et al. Missed diagnoses in patients with upper gastrointestinal cancers. Endoscopy. 2004;36:874e9.
11. Fitzgerald RC, Saeed IT, Khoo D, et al. Rigorous surveillance protocol increases detection of curable cancers associated with Barrett's esophagus. Dig Dis Sci. 2001;46:1892e8.
12. Bramble MG, Suvakovic Z, Hungin AP. Detection of upper gastrointestinal cancer in patients taking antisecretory therapy prior to gastroscopy. Gut. 2000;46:464e7.
13. Meister T, Heinzow HS, et al. Miniprobe endoscopic ultrasound accurately stages esophageal cancer and guides therapeutic decisions in the era of neoadjuvant therapy: results of a multicenter cohort analysis. Surg Endosc. 2013;27(8):2813–9.
14. Catalano MF, Sivak Jr MV, Rice T, et al. Endosonographic features predictive of lymph node metastasis. Gastrointest Endosc. 1994;40:442e6.
15. Vazquez-Sequeiros E, Norton ID, Clain JE, et al. Impact of EUS-guided fine-needle aspiration on lymph node staging in patients with esophageal carcinoma. Gastrointest Endosc. 2001;53:751e7.13. Catalano MF, Sivak MV Jr, Rice T, et al. Endosonographic features predictive of lymph node metastasis. Gastrointest Endosc. 1994;40:442e6.
16. Bhandari S, Shim CS, Kim JH, et al. Usefulness of three-dimensional, multidetector row CT (virtual gastroscopy and multiplanar reconstruction) in the evaluation of gastric cancer: a

comparison with conventional endoscopy, EUS, and histopathology. Gastrointest Endosc. 2004;59:619e26.

17. Fukuya T, Honda H, Kaneko K, et al. Efficacy of helical CT in T-staging of gastric cancer. J Comput Assist Tomogr. 1997;21:73e81.

18. Yajima K, et al. Clinical and diagnostic significance of preoperative computed tomography findings of ascites in patients with advanced gastric cancer. Am J Surg. 2006;192(2):185–90.

19. Purandare NC, et al. Incremental value of 18F-FDG PET/CT in therapeutic decision-making of potentially curable esophageal adenocarcinoma. Nucl Mcd Commun. 2014;35(8):864–9.

20. Bruzzi JF, et al. PET/CT of esophageal cancer: its role in clinical management. Radiographics. 2007;27(6):1635–52.

21. Edge S, et al. AJCC Cancer Staging Manual. 7th ed. New York, NY: Springer, 2010, pp 129–35.

Pathology of Oesophageal Cancer and Gastric Cancer

2

Nilu Wijesuriya

Contents

2.1 Introduction

Squamous cell carcinoma, adenocarcinoma and small cell carcinoma comprise the three most frequent histological subtypes of primary carcinomas arising in the upper gastrointestinal (UGI) tract [1, 2]. The two former subtypes, which account for the majority, are described in more detail.

2.2 Oesophageal Cancer

The histological classification of tumours of the oesophagus, according to the WHO, is shown in Table 2.1. Of these, squamous cell carcinoma and adenocarcinoma are the most common subtypes.

N. Wijesuriya
Cellular Pathology, Barts Health NHS Trust, London, UK
e-mail: niluchampika@doctors.org.uk

© Springer International Publishing Switzerland 2016
T.A. Szyszko (ed.), *PET/CT in Oesophageal and Gastric Cancer*, Clinicians' Guides
to Radionuclide Hybrid Imaging, DOI 10.1007/978-3-319-29240-3_2

Table 2.1 WHO classification of tumours of the oesophagus [1]

Epithelial tumours	Mesenchymal tumours
Premalignant lesions	Granular cell tumour
Low-grade squamous dysplasia	Haemangioma
High-grade squamous dysplasia	Leiomyoma
Low-grade glandular dysplasia	Lipoma
High-grade glandular dysplasia	Gastrointestinal stromal tumour (GIST)
	Kaposi sarcoma
Carcinoma	Leiomyosarcoma
Squamous cell carcinoma	Melanoma
Adenocarcinoma	Rhabdomyosarcoma
Adenoid cystic carcinoma	Synovial sarcoma
Adenosquamous carcinoma	
Basaloid squamous cell carcinoma	
Mucoepidermoid carcinoma	
Spindle cell (squamous) carcinoma	*Lymphomas*
Verrucous (squamous) carcinoma	
Undifferentiated carcinoma	
Neuroendocrine neoplasms	*Secondary/metastatic tumours*
Neuroendocrine tumour (NET) (grades 1 and 2)	
Large-cell neuroendocrine carcinoma	
Small cell neuroendocrine carcinoma	
Mixed adenoneuroendocrine carcinoma	

2.2.1 Squamous Cell Carcinoma (SCC)

A malignant epithelial neoplasm derived from the lining squamous epithelium and therefore showing squamous cell differentiation. Most arise in the middle third of the organ followed by the lower and upper thirds, respectively [1].

Macroscopy
Grossly, tumours can show protruding, ulcerative or infiltrative appearances depending on the depth of invasion [3].

Microscopy
SCC is thought to arise from precursor intraepithelial neoplasia in which the squamous epithelial lining shows dysplasia, but no breach of the basement membrane. Invasion is confirmed by penetration across the epithelial basement membrane into the lamina propria. Invasive carcinoma is characterised by keratinocyte-like cells which show atypical nuclear features and deeply eosinophilic cytoplasm [1, 2]. The likelihood of invasion of lymphatic channels and intramural veins increases with the depth of penetration across the oesophageal wall. Extension into the adventitia can lead to the involvement of adjacent soft tissue and organs.

Histological grading into well-differentiated, moderately differentiated and poorly differentiated SCCs depends upon mitotic activity, nuclear atypia and extent

Fig. 2.1 Moderately differentiated SCC invading the muscularis propria characterised by neoplastic islands of squamous epithelium showing central keratinisation (*arrow*)

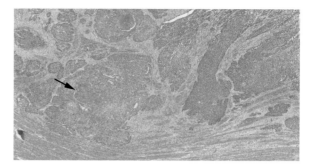

of squamous differentiation, although its significance with regard to prognostication divides opinion [4]. Well-differentiated tumours show more prominent keratinisation with the formation of squamous pearls in comparison to poorly differentiated tumours which can show only occasional keratinised cells.

Variants of SCC include basaloid SCC, verrucous carcinoma and spindle cell squamous carcinoma [1, 2] (Fig. 2.1).

Immunohistochemistry
Tumour cells show cytoplasmic and membranous positivity for high-molecular-weight keratins such as LP34 and CK5/6 and nuclear positivity for the transcription protein p63 [5]. Immunohistochemistry can be particularly useful in detecting residual tumour in resection specimens following neoadjuvant treatment which may otherwise not be evident on routine H + E staining.

Molecular Pathology
TP53 gene mutations are sometimes seen in precursor lesions [1, 2], and 20–40 % of SCCs can show amplification of cyclin D1 [6].

2.2.2 Adenocarcinoma

A malignant epithelial neoplasm characterised by glandular differentiation and mucin production. Most arise in the lower oesophagus [1, 2], and the majority are associated with intestinal metaplasia or Barrett's oesophagus. The latter is the replacement of squamous epithelium of the oesophagus by columnar-lined epithelium due to repetitive injury usually as a result of chronic gastro-oesophageal reflux disease [1, 7, 8].

Macroscopy
Tumours can be flat and ulcerated or polypoid and fungating [1].

Microscopy
Progression from Barrett's oesophagus to adenocarcinoma is a multistep process with the development of increasing architectural and cytological atypia or dysplasia

Fig. 2.2 Moderately differentiated adenocarcinoma of the oesophagus arising on a background Barrett's oesophagus with high-grade dysplasia. A small residual island of squamous epithelium is also noted (*arrow*)

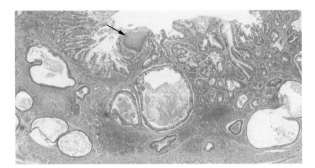

Fig. 2.3 Poorly differentiated adenocarcinoma of the oesophagus with a solid growth pattern. Adjacent Barrett's oesophagus with high-grade dysplasia is also seen (*arrow*)

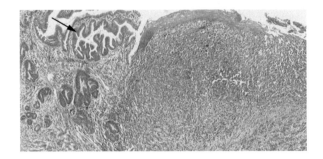

[1, 2]. Adenocarcinomas are classified according to the gastric cancer classification (see later), and most invasive tumours are of intestinal type with tubular and papillary growth patterns although diffuse patterns with signet-ring cells are also encountered [1, 2]. As with SCC, the likelihood of lymphovascular invasion and lymph node metastases increases with the depth of penetration. Histological grade divides tumours into well-differentiated, moderately differentiated or poorly differentiated forms with the latter showing more solid growth patterns and poorly formed glandular structures (Figs. 2.2 and 2.3).

Special Stains and Immunohistochemistry
Histochemical stains such as periodic acid-Schiff diastase (PASD) can be used to highlight mucin production by tumour cells. The usual immunohistochemical profile is that of positivity for CK7 and negativity for CK20 [5].

Molecular Pathology
A variety of tumour suppressor genes, oncogenes and receptors have been implicated in the progression of oesophageal adenocarcinoma including mutations in *TP53*, *KRAS* and *ERBB2* [9–11].

2.3   Gastric Carcinoma

The WHO classification of tumours of the stomach is shown in Table 2.2. Of these, adenocarcinoma accounts for the majority of primary tumours.

Table 2.2 WHO classification of the tumours of the stomach [1]

Epithelial tumours	Mesenchymal tumours
Premalignant lesions	Glomus tumour
Adenoma	Granular cell tumour
Low-grade dysplasia	Leiomyoma
High-grade dysplasia	Plexiform fibromyxoma
	Schwannoma
Carcinoma	Inflammatory myofibroblastic tumour
Adenocarcinoma	Gastrointestinal stromal tumour (GIST)
Adenosquamous carcinoma	Kaposi sarcoma
Carcinoma with lymphoid stroma	Leiomyosarcoma
Hepatoid adenocarcinoma	Synovial sarcoma
Squamous cell carcinoma	
Undifferentiated carcinoma	
Neuroendocrine neoplasms	*Lymphomas*
Neuroendocrine tumours (NET) (grades 1 and 2)	
Large-cell neuroendocrine carcinoma	
Small cell neuroendocrine carcinoma	
Mixed adenoneuroendocrine carcinoma	*Secondary/metastatic tumours*
EC cell, serotonin-producing NET	
Gastrin-producing NET	

Table 2.3 Lauren and WHO classification for gastric adenocarcinoma

Lauren classification	WHO classification
Intestinal type	Tubular adenocarcinoma
	Papillary adenocarcinoma
Diffuse type	Mucinous adenocarcinoma
	Poorly cohesive carcinoma
Mixed	Mixed adenocarcinoma

Macroscopy

The gross appearance varies according to the depth of invasion. Early gastric carcinoma (those confined to the mucosa and submucosa) can show protruded, elevated, flat, depressed and excavated patterns [2, 12]. Advanced tumours are described according to the Borrmann classification which recognises polypoid, fungating, ulcerated and infiltrative types [1, 2].

Microscopy

As is the case elsewhere in the UGI tract, the development of gastric adenocarcinoma may be preceded by a variety of precancerous lesions. Chronic atrophic gastritis (due to *Helicobacter pylori* infection and autoimmune gastritis) and intestinal metaplasia are recognised risk factors for the development of dysplasia and carcinoma [2, 13].

A number of histological classifications exist for gastric adenocarcinoma of which the Lauren and WHO classifications are the most widely recognised and used [2, 14, 15] (Table 2.3). Figure 2.4 demonstrates a moderately differentiated gastric adenocarcinoma (Lauren intestinal type) and Fig. 2.5 a poorly differentiated gastric adenocarcinoma (Lauren diffuse type).

Fig. 2.4 Demonstrates a
moderately differentiated
gastric adenocarcinoma
(Lauren intestinal type)
with the formation of
recognisable neoplastic
glands

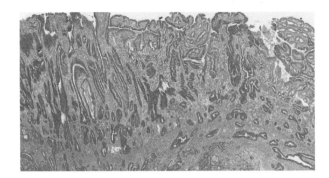

Fig. 2.5 Poorly
differentiated gastric
adenocarcinoma (Lauren
diffuse type) with poorly
cohesive tumour cells
showing classic signet-ring
cell morphology (*arrow*)

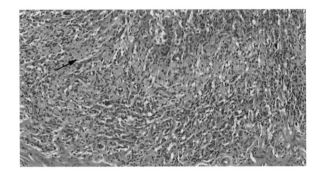

Tumour spread can occur via lymphatic and haematogenous routes or by direct extension across the wall to involve adjacent organs. Peritoneal extension is also seen, especially with diffuse subtypes [1, 2].

Immunohistochemistry

Gastric adenocarcinomas show strong positivity for a number of cytokeratins, and approximately 50 % are strongly positive for CK7 in a diffuse or patchy pattern. The CK7/CK20 staining patterns can be quite variable and not always helpful in distinguishing from other UGI tract adenocarcinomas [5]. The HER2 status as assessed by immunohistochemistry can be helpful in certain cases of advanced gastric cancer for targeted therapy [16].

Molecular Pathology

Different genetic pathways have been described for various histological subtypes of gastric adenocarcinoma including mutations in oncogenes, tumour suppressor genes and DNA mismatch genes [1, 2].

2.4   Adenocarcinomas of the Gastro-oesophageal Junction (GOJ)

Adenocarcinomas which straddle the GOJ can pose problems with regard to localisation and therefore pathological staging. A widely used classification to overcome this conundrum is that proposed by Siewert and Stein in which adenocarcinomas of the GOJ are defined as tumours with an epicentre within 5 cm of the anatomical cardia [2, 17]. In this classification, adenocarcinomas involving the GOJ are separated into three subtypes: type 1 (distal oesophagus) as those arising 1–5 cm above the GOJ, type 2 (true carcinoma of the cardia) and type 3 (subcardial gastric carcinoma) as those 2–5 cm below the GOJ. The GOJ is defined by the proximal limits of the gastric rugal folds.

SCCs involving the GOJ are regarded as those arising in the distal oesophagus even if tumours cross the junction to involve the proximal stomach [1].

Keypoints
- The three most frequent histological subtypes of primary carcinomas arising in the upper gastrointestinal (UGI) tract include squamous cell carcinoma, adenocarcinoma and small cell carcinoma.
- Most SCCs of oesophagus arise in the middle third of the organ followed by the lower and upper thirds, respectively.
- Microscopic invasion is confirmed by penetration across the epithelial basement membrane into the lamina propria.
- Extension into the adventitia can lead to the involvement of adjacent soft tissue and organs.
- Histological grading into well-differentiated, moderately differentiated and poorly differentiated SCCs depends upon mitotic activity, nuclear atypia and extent of squamous differentiation.
- Immunohistochemistry can be particularly useful in detecting residual tumour in resection specimens following neoadjuvant treatment.
- Most adenocarcinomas arise in the lower oesophagus, and the majority are associated with intestinal metaplasia or Barrett's oesophagus.
- Adenocarcinoma accounts for the majority of primary tumours of the stomach.
- Development of gastric adenocarcinoma may be preceded by a variety of precancerous lesions.
- Gastric tumour spread can occur via lymphatic and haematogenous routes or by direct extension across the wall to involve adjacent organs.

References

1. Bosman FT, Carneiro F, Hruban RH, Theise ND, editors. World Health Organisation classification of tumours of the digestive system. 4th ed. Lyon: IARC press; 2010.
2. Sarbia M, Becker KF, Höfler H. Pathology of upper gastrointestinal malignancies. Semin Oncol. 2004;31(4):465–75.
3. Japan Esophageal Society. Japanese classification of esophageal cancer, 10th edition: part 1. Esophagus. 2009;6:1–25.
4. Sarbia M, Bittinger F, Porschen R, et al. Prognostic value of histopathologic parameters of esophageal squamous cell carcinoma. Cancer. 1995;76(6):922–7.
5. Neal S, Bosler D. Immunohistochemistry of the gastrointestinal tract, pancreas, bile ducts, gallbladder and liver. In: Dabbs DJ, editor. From diagnostic immunohistochemistry. 2nd ed. New York: Churchill Livingstone; 2006.
6. Jiang W, Zhang YJ, Kahn SM, et al. Altered expression of the cyclin D1 and the retinoblastoma genes in human esophageal cancer. Proc Natl Acad Sci U S A. 1993;90(19):9026–30.
7. Lagergren J. Adenocarcinoma of the oesophagus: what exactly is the size of the problem and who is at risk? Gut. 2005;54(1):1–5.
8. Wild CP, Hardie LJ. Reflux, Barrett's oesophagus and adenocarcinoma: burning questions. Nat Rev Cancer. 2003;3(9):676–84.
9. Sato F, Meltzer SJ. CpG island hypermethylation in progression of esophageal and gastric cancer. Cancer. 2006;106(3):483–93.
10. Sommerer F, Vieth M, Markwarth A, et al. Mutations of BRAF and KRAS2 in the development of Barrett's adenocarcinoma. Oncogene. 2004;23(2):554–8.
11. Walch A, Specht K, Braselmann H, et al. Coamplification and coexpression of GRB7 and ERBB2 is found in high grade intraepithelial neoplasia and in invasive Barrett's carcinoma. Int J Cancer. 2004;112(5):747–53.
12. Ohta H, Noguchi Y, Takagi K, et al. Early gastric carcinoma with special reference to macroscopic classification. Cancer. 1987;60(5):1099–106.
13. Correa P, Piazuelo MB. The gastric precancerous cascade. J Dig Dis. 2012;13(1):2–9.
14. Berlth F, Bollschweiler E, Drebber U, et al. Pathohistological classification systems in gastric cancer: diagnostic relevance and prognostic value. World J Gastroenterol. 2014;20(19):5679–84.
15. Lauren P. The two histological main types of gastric carcinoma: diffuse and so-called intestinal-type carcinoma. An attempt at a histo-clinical classification. Acta Pathol Scand. 1965;64:31–49.
16. Boku N. HER2-positive gastric cancer. Gastric Cancer. 2014;17:1–12.
17. Siewert JR, Stein H. Classification of adenocarcinoma of the oesophago-gastric junction. Br J Cancer. 1998;85:1457–9.

Management of Oesophageal and Gastric Cancers

3

David Propper and Kathryn Hawkesford

Contents

3.1 Oesophageal Cancer

Oesophageal cancer aetiologically, therapeutically and prognostically should be divided into two common histological types, rather than considered together, although many of the treatments overlap. Squamous cancers can affect the entire oesophagus, whereas adenocarcinomas are confined to the distal oesophagus and gastro-oesophageal junction. Most tumours present at stage T3 or greater and/or are node positive, and cure with multimodality therapy is only around 15 %.

D. Propper (✉)
Barts Cancer Institute, Queen Mary University of London, London, UK
e-mail: d.j.propper@qmul.ac.uk

K. Hawkesford
Department of Medical Oncology, Barts Health NHS Trust, London, UK

© Springer International Publishing Switzerland 2016
T.A. Szyszko (ed.), *PET/CT in Oesophageal and Gastric Cancer*, Clinicians' Guides to Radionuclide Hybrid Imaging, DOI 10.1007/978-3-319-29240-3_3

17

Preoperative Staging

As discussed in Chap. 1, staging of local disease for depth of invasion (T stage) or N stage is best achieved by endoscopic ultrasonography (EUS) and CT scanning for distant disease. FDG-PET/CT scanning can upstage tumours and is a standard practice. In development is the use of FDG-PET/CT scanning at presentation and after treatment as a guide to prognosis [1].

3.2 Oesophageal Cancer Treatment

3.2.1 Curative

Early tumours, namely, those confined to the mucosa (T1a), can be treated by endoscopic mucosal resection (EMR), of which there is considerable experience, or by ablative modalities, including photodynamic therapy (PDT), argon plasma coagulation (APC), radiofrequency ablation (RFA) and laser therapy where there is less data [2]. More advanced tumours need surgical or combined modality treatments.

Squamous Carcinoma

Oesophageal squamous carcinoma typically has a worse prognosis compared to adenocarcinoma. It has a tendency to spread early. Because of this, it is common practice to consider only T1–T2 stage tumours for initial surgery. T3 and T4 tumours have often spread either submucosally or along lymphatics so that surgery at this stage is rarely curative [3]. Hence affected patients are treated with chemoradiotherapy. The effects of chemoradiotherapy and surgery on survival rates are similar [4], although significant number of tumours do not respond fully to chemoradiotherapy. These patients are considered for salvage surgery.

Adenocarcinoma

Patients with T2 N0 disease or less proceed directly to surgery. Patients with more advanced or with nodal disease receive preoperative chemotherapy, typically two to three cycles of a platinum plus fluoropyrimidine-containing regimen. This is associated with an absolute survival benefit at 5 years of at least 6 % [5, 6]. Whether combined chemoradiotherapy before surgery for adenocarcinoma is superior to chemotherapy is controversial. There have been no adequate comparisons between the two modalities. A recent Cochrane review suggested a trend to greater survival for chemoradiotherapy as compared to chemotherapy in oesophageal and oesophagogastric junction tumours [7].

3.2.2 Palliative Therapies

Local therapies are directed at relieving obstruction or other local symptoms. This typically involves either stenting or radiotherapy. Systematic therapies comprise the same chemotherapy regimens as used in gastric cancer and are discussed below.

3.3   Gastric Cancer

Staging and Preoperative Evaluation
The TNM staging for gastric cancer is similar to oesophageal carcinoma. Preoperative staging is most effectively done by CT scans of the chest, abdomen and pelvis. Although CT is not specifically accurate for assessing the depth of tumour invasion of the stomach wall or regional nodal involvement, it is useful for staging distant spread. Staging laparoscopy is standard for any medically fit patient with beyond a T1 tumour. These modalities obviate the role of EUS, which is not routine in many centres unless the tumour involves the oesophagogastric junction.

The role of FDG-PET/CT in the preoperative staging of gastric adenocarcinoma is evolving. Signet-ring carcinomas are not FDG avid [8], and the sensitivity of FDG-PET for peritoneal carcinomatosis is only approximately 50 % [9]. Hence PET scanning is not as utilised as it is for oesophageal cancer, although significant upstaging rates of approximately 10 % have been described in patients with $\geq$ T3 or $\geq$ N1 disease [10].

3.4   Gastric Cancer Treatment

EMR is feasible for early gastric cancers (T1a) if well differentiated, $\leq$ 2 cm, and not ulcerated [11]. Surgery alone is recommended for any < T2 N0 disease.

3.4.1   Chemotherapy

Patients with more advanced stages should receive preoperative adjuvant chemotherapy. This is associated with an absolute survival increase of 9 % at 5 years [7]. Typically this comprises three cycles of a platinum and fluoropyrimidine combination with or without epirubicin. Postoperative adjuvant chemotherapy also reduces recurrence rates [12]; however, frequently there is considerable delay in patients receiving postoperative treatment, and many fail to complete. Hence preoperative chemotherapy is the preferred option.

3.4.1.1 Palliative Chemotherapy
Systemic chemotherapy is used for inoperable or metastatic oesophagogastric cancer.

Meta-analysis comparing chemotherapy to the best supportive care shows an improvement in median survival from 4.3 to 11 months [13]. Fluoropyrimidine-/platinum-containing or other doublet regimens are associated with improved survival in comparison to single-agent fluoropyrimidine regimens [13].

In general, response rates to primary chemotherapy are between 35 and 50 % with a further significant proportion achieving disease stabilisation. There is no consensus on which regimen to use as first-line treatment. Commonly used regimens include epirubicin, oxaliplatin and capecitabine (EOX) and docetaxel, cisplatin, and infusional 5-FU (DCF) combinations. These are relatively toxic regimens, particularly DCF [14], and since combination regimens probably only modestly improve survival compared to single-agent regimens, it is appropriate to use single-agent regimens in elderly patients or those with reduced performance status.

Second-line chemotherapy can modestly (by around 8 weeks) prolong survival compared to the best supportive care, and both irinotecan and docetaxel have efficacy, probably with improved quality of life [15, 16].

3.4.2   Biological Agents

There is a limited place for biological agents. The addition of the HER2-targeted antibody trastuzumab in patients with oesophagogastric adenocarcinomas expressing HER2 (about 20 % of tumours) [17] improved response rates and overall survival by approximately 10 weeks in patient receiving first-line combination of platinum and fluoropyrimidine chemotherapy [18].

Recently, ramucirumab, a monoclonal antibody which binds VEGFR-2, was reported to produce a modest survival prolongation (approximately 6–8 weeks) in patients with previously treated oesophagogastric adenocarcinoma [19].

Key Points

- Early tumours confined to the mucosa (T1a) can be treated by endoscopic mucosal resection (EMR) or by ablative modalities (PDT, APC, RFA) and laser therapy.
- More advanced tumours need surgical or combined modality treatments.
- Oesophageal squamous carcinoma has a worse prognosis compared to adenocarcinoma.
- Oesophageal squamous carcinoma: Only stages T1 and T2 are considered for initial surgery and T3/T4 stages for chemoradiotherapy.
- The role of FDG-PET/CT in the preoperative staging of gastric adenocarcinoma is evolving.
- EMR is feasible for early gastric cancers (T1a) if well differentiated, ≤ 2 cm, and not ulcerated [11]. Surgery alone is recommended for any $<$T2 N0 disease.
- Patients with more advanced gastric cancer stages should receive preoperative adjuvant chemotherapy.
- Systemic chemotherapy is used for inoperable or metastatic oesophagogastric cancer.
- There is a limited place for biological agents.

References

1. Kwee RM. Prediction of tumor response to neoadjuvant therapy in patients with esophageal cancer with use of 18F FDG PET: a systematic review. Radiology. 2010;254(3):707–17.
2. Prasad GA, Wu TT, Wigle DA, et al. Endoscopic and surgical treatment of mucosal (T1a) esophageal adenocarcinoma in Barrett's esophagus. Gastroenterology. 2009;137(3):815–23.
3. Siewert JR, Ott K. Are squamous and adenocarcinomas of the esophagus the same disease? Semin Radiat Oncol. 2007;17(1):38–44.
4. Allum WH, Blazeby JM, Griffin SM, et al. Guidelines for the management of oesophageal and gastric cancer. Gut. 2011;60(11):1449–72.
5. Allum WH, Stenning SP, Bancewicz J, et al. Long-term results of a randomized trial of surgery with or without preoperative chemotherapy in esophageal cancer. J Clin Oncol. 2009;27(30):5062–7.
6. Ychou M, Boige V, Pignon JP, et al. Perioperative chemotherapy compared with surgery alone for resectable gastroesophageal adenocarcinoma: an FNCLCC and FFCD multicenter phase III trial. J Clin Oncol. 2011;29(13):1715–21.
7. Ronellenfitsch U, Schwarzbach M, Hofheinz R, et al. Perioperative chemo(radio)therapy versus primary surgery for resectable adenocarcinoma of the stomach, gastroesophageal junction, and lower esophagus. Cochrane Database Syst Rev. 2013;5:CD008107.
8. Stahl A, Ott K, Weber WA, et al. FDG PET imaging of locally advanced gastric carcinomas: correlation with endoscopic and histopathological findings. Eur J Nucl Med Mol Imaging. 2003;30(2):288–95.
9. Yoshioka T, Yamaguchi K, Kubota K, et al. Evaluation of 18F-FDG PET in patients with advanced, metastatic, or recurrent gastric cancer. J Nucl Med. 2003;44(5):690–9.
10. Smyth E, Schoder H, Strong VE, et al. A prospective evaluation of the utility of 2-deoxy-2-[(18) F]fluoro-D-glucose positron emission tomography and computed tomography in staging locally advanced gastric cancer. Cancer. 2012;118(22):5481–8.
11. Tada M, Tanaka Y, Matsuo N, et al. Mucosectomy for gastric cancer: current status in Japan. J Gastroenterol Hepatol. 2000;15(Suppl):D98–102.
12. Bang YJ, Kim YW, Yang HK, et al. Adjuvant capecitabine and oxaliplatin for gastric cancer after D2 gastrectomy (CLASSIC): a phase 3 open-label, randomised controlled trial. Lancet. 2012;379(9813):315–21.
13. Wagner AD, Unverzagt S, Grothe W, et al. Chemotherapy for advanced gastric cancer. Cochrane Database Syst Rev. 2010;(3):CD004064.
14. Van Cutsem E, Moiseyenko VM, Tjulandin S, et al. Phase III study of docetaxel and cisplatin plus fluorouracil compared with cisplatin and fluorouracil as first-line therapy for advanced gastric cancer: a report of the V325 Study Group. J Clin Oncol. 2006;24(31):4991–7.
15. Kang JH, Lee SI, do Lim H, et al. Salvage chemotherapy for pretreated gastric cancer: a randomized phase III trial comparing chemotherapy plus best supportive care with best supportive care alone. J Clin Oncol. 2012;30(13):1513–8.
16. Park SH, Lee WK, Chung M, et al. Quality of life in patients with advanced gastric cancer treated with second-line chemotherapy. Cancer Chemother Pharmacol. 2006;57(3):289–94.
17. Tanner M, Hollmen M, Junttila TT, et al. Amplification of HER-2 in gastric carcinoma: association with Topoisomerase II alpha gene amplification, intestinal type, poor prognosis and sensitivity to trastuzumab. Ann Oncol. 2005;16(2):273–8.
18. Bang YJ, Van Cutsem E, Feyereislova A, et al. Trastuzumab in combination with chemotherapy versus chemotherapy alone for treatment of HER2-positive advanced gastric or gastro-oesophageal junction cancer (ToGA): a phase 3, open-label, randomised controlled trial. Lancet. 2010;376(9742):687–97.
19. Fuchs CS, Tomasek J, Yong CJ, et al. Ramucirumab monotherapy for previously treated advanced gastric or gastro-oesophageal junction adenocarcinoma (REGARD): an international, randomised, multicentre, placebo-controlled, phase 3 trial. Lancet. 2014;383(9911):31–9.

Radiological Imaging in Oesophageal and Gastric Cancers

4

Ayshea Hameeduddin

Contents

4.1 Introduction

Imaging modalities used to assess carcinoma of the oesophagus and stomach include barium studies, endoscopic ultrasound (EUS), multi-detector CT (MDCT), magnetic resonance imaging (MRI) and PET-CT (see separate chapter). Historically, patients who presented with dysphagia were frequently referred for a barium swallow study if an irregular stricture was identified they proceeded to endoscopy for diagnosis. Assessment of the stomach with barium required a double-contrast study with contrast and air to detect and localise a gastric tumour; however due to advances in endoscopy, EUS and MDCT, the use of barium studies has declined [1].

A. Hameeduddin
Radiology and Nuclear Medicine, Barts Health NHS Trust, London, UK
e-mail: aysheah@googlemail.com; Ayshea.Hameeduddin@bartshealth.nhs.uk

© Springer International Publishing Switzerland 2016   23
T.A. Szyszko (ed.), *PET/CT in Oesophageal and Gastric Cancer*, Clinicians' Guides
to Radionuclide Hybrid Imaging, DOI 10.1007/978-3-319-29240-3_4

EUS is currently the preferred modality in diagnosis of both oesophageal and gastric carcinomas, allowing assessment of the depth of tumour invasion and concurrent histological diagnosis. MDCT is the mainstay of pretreatment staging, radiotherapy planning, response assessment and surveillance imaging. MRI has a limited role in staging due to artefacts from cardiorespiratory motion in the thorax and abdomen; although there have been technical advances allowing faster imaging acquisitions, availability, economic and patient comfort factors remain sufficient barriers to widespread use.

4.2   Diagnosis and Staging

A multimodality imaging approach is used to accurately assess tumours according to the clinical TNM staging system which allows stratification of patients to optimal therapeutic pathways. Each imaging modality has advantages and limitations summarised in Table 4.1.

4.2.1   T Stage

EUS is considered the most accurate modality for diagnosis and assessing the depth of tumour invasion as it allows differentiation of the five layers of the oesophageal and gastric wall and therefore the delineation of T1, T2 and T3 tumours (see Fig. 4.1). Simultaneous biopsies allow for histological correlation [1–3]. With technical advances in endoscopic ultrasound probes, the differentiation between T1m (mucosal) and T1sm (submucosal) oesophageal tumours is possible. This has important clinical implications in the choice of local ablative therapy or endoscopic mucosal resection [4]. Limitations to EUS include difficulty in assessment of

Table 4.1 Summary of advantages and limitations

Modality	Advantages	Limitations
EUS	Allows accurate assessment of depth of tumour (T stage)	Cannot assess distant metastases
		Operator dependent
	Can sample tumour and local lymph nodes	Risk of perforation
		Stenotic tumours difficult to assess
	Higher accuracy than CT	May overstage post treatment
CT	Assessment of T4 disease	Cannot assess depth of tumour invasion
	3D-reformats allow both surgical and radiotherapy planning	Lymph node assessment limited due to size criteria
	Detection of suspicious non-regional lymph nodes	Cannot differentiate viable tumour from fibrosis post treatment
	Excellent at assessing metastatic disease	
MRI	Non-ionising radiation	Motion artefact degrades images
		Not widely available
		Expensive

Fig. 4.1 Endoscopic ultrasound image of an oesophageal tumour between the callipers marked *D1* which measured 1.5 cm. There is loss of the normal alternating hypo- and hyperechoic layers of the oesophageal wall and a bulge in the left lateral wall corresponding to a T3 tumour. Note the normal appearances of the layers of the oesophageal wall

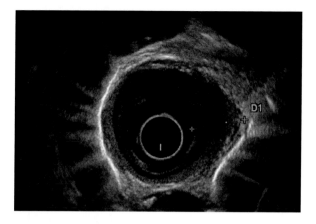

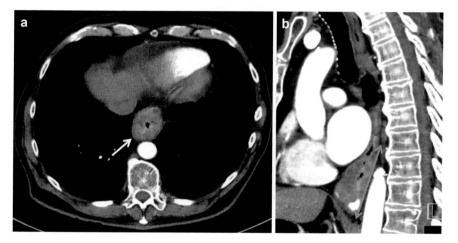

Fig. 4.2 (**a**) Axial contrast-enhanced CT image showing circumferential thickening of the lower third of the oesophagus consistent with a T3 tumour (*white arrow*). (**b**) Sagittal reconstruction showing the craniocaudal length of the tumour which is useful for surgical planning (*blue arrow*)

stenotic tumours as the probe cannot pass through the lumen and there is a risk of perforation [5].

MDCT has a limited role in the assessment of T1 and T2 tumours due to the difficulty in differentiating layers of the bowel wall and has been shown to have poorer sensitivity in detecting the primary tumour in both oesophageal and gastric carcinomas compared to EUS [2, 3, 6]. To optimise detection of tumours on CT, the stomach should be distended with oral contrast (barium or water) [1]. The normal thickness of the oesophageal wall is less than 3 mm when distended, a thickness greater than 5 mm is considered abnormal (see Fig. 4.2) [7].

In a systematic review by Kwee et al. EUS, MDCT and MRI had equivocal results in diagnostic accuracy in T staging of gastric carcinoma, although few MRI studies were available and the authors concluded that EUS was superior [3].

Table 4.2 CT criteria for diagnosing mediastinal invasion

Loss of fat plane between the tumour and adjacent structures in the mediastinum

Displacement or indentation of other mediastinal structures

Aortic invasion suggested if >90° of the aorta is in contact with the tumour or if there is obliteration of the triangular fat space between the oesophagus, aorta and spine adjacent to the primary tumour

Tracheobronchial fistula

Pericardial invasion suspected if thickening of the pericardium, pericardial effusion, loss of pericardial fat plane between the heart and pericardium

In oesophageal carcinoma, an important role of MDCT is differentiating T4a and T4b tumours and therefore selecting patients for surgery. T4a tumours invade the pleura, pericardium or diaphragm and are resectable, whereas T4b tumours are inoperable invading the trachea, aorta or bone [6]. The CT criteria for diagnosing mediastinal invasion are summarised in Table 4.2.

The ability to reformat images in axial, coronal and sagittal planes can aid surgical planning in the patients selected for curative resection. The upper resection margin should be 8–10 cm above the tumour and the lower margin 5 cm below the tumour [8].

4.2.2 N Stage

Lymph node involvement is a predictor of survival, and therefore distinguishing loco-regional lymph nodes from distant non-regional nodal metastases is important for deciding on the best management options. In patients with oesophageal carcinoma, surgery is an option for loco-regional nodal involvement, whereas distant nodes in the retroperitoneum or mid-neck are considered M1 disease and a contraindication to surgery [6].

EUS with fine-needle aspiration is superior to CT in detecting regional lymph node involvement. EUS uses both size criteria and the internal echogenicity of the lymph nodes to assess for disease involvement and has a published accuracy of 89 % compared to 75 % for CT [9]. The main limitation of CT is that pathological lymph nodes are identified based on size criteria. Lymph nodes are required to be greater than 10 mm in short axis in the chest and abdomen, over 5 mm in the supraclavicular fossa and over 6 mm retrocrural regions to be identified as abnormal [6]. A difficulty in gastric carcinoma is that hepatoduodenal lymph nodes are considered M1 disease but can be difficult to differentiate from regional common hepatic lymph nodes [1].

CT has better accuracy than EUS in identifying mediastinal lymph nodes and also nodes that are outside of the normal surgical field, which would not normally be resected. Using 3D CT reformats can help to distinguish lymph nodes from perigastric and oesophageal vessels (see Fig. 4.3).

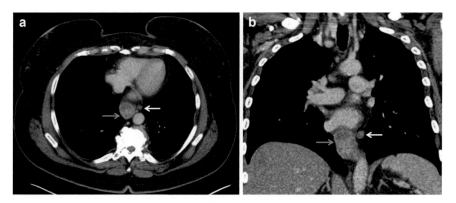

Fig. 4.3 Contrast-enhanced axial (**a**) and coronal (**b**) CT reformats showing a perioesophageal lymph node (*white arrows*); note how the node is more readily identifiable in the coronal plane and easily distinguished from vessels. The oesophageal tumour is marked with the *blue arrows*

Table 4.3   Signs of peritoneal disease on CT [9]

Ascites
Soft tissue nodules or plaques on the peritoneal surface
Thickening of the peritoneal reflections
Small bowel wall thickening
Intra-abdominal fat stranding
Peritoneal enhancement

4.2.3   M Stage

The mainstay of evaluation of distant metastatic disease is with contrast-enhanced MDCT. The commonest sites of spread are the lungs, liver, bone and adrenal glands. Pulmonary metastases appear as round soft tissue density lesions of varying size throughout the lung parenchyma, and liver metastases are usually hypoattenuating and ill defined. Bone metastases may be destructive or sclerotic. In gastric carcinoma the presence of ascites is the most important factor to predict peritoneal carcinomatosis [1]. Signs of peritoneal disease on CT are summarised in Table 4.3. Identifying distant disease immediately streamlines patients into systemic or palliative treatment options (Fig. 4.4).

4.3   Response Assessment

Both EUS and MDCT are routinely used in the post-treatment assessment of disease response; however, both modalities have limitations. After chemoradiotherapy, it is difficult to distinguish fibrosis, necrosis and inflammatory changes from residual tumour, and there is a tendency to overstage on EUS [10]. Furthermore, EUS is not possible in up to 6 % of patients who develop luminal stenosis post-treatment [11].

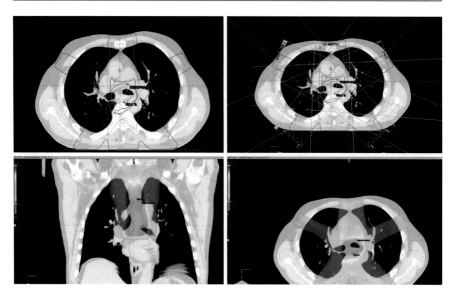

Fig. 4.4 Multiplanar axial and coronal CT images showing intensity-modulated radiation therapy (IMRT) planning images

CT cannot differentiate oesophageal or gastric wall thickening due to viable tumour from inflammatory changes. If there has been a reduction in size of the primary tumour, associated nodal disease and no evidence of new sites of disease on CT, then surgery may be considered.

4.4   Radiotherapy Planning

Multiplanar CT allows the planning of radiotherapy by allowing the delineation of the primary tumour and regional lymph nodes with the aim of minimising radiation to the adjacent normal structures.

Conclusion

Accurate radiological assessment of oesophageal and gastric carcinomas is vital to stratify patients according to the TNM classification into appropriate treatment options. A multimodality approach is used with the mainstay of assessment EUS and MDCT. EUS is superior to CT in T staging and N staging of locoregional disease, whereas CT has a role in the assessment of distant nodal and M staging of disease. Furthermore, sophisticated radiotherapy treatments are planned on multiplanar CT reformats. Both EUS and CT have limitations concerning response assessment, and FDG-PET has emerged as a useful modality in this setting.

Key Points
- Accurate radiological assessment of oesophageal and gastric carcinomas is vital to stratify patients.
- Imaging modalities used in the assessment of oesophageal and stomach cancers include barium studies, EUS, MDCT, MRI and PET-CT.
- MDCT is the mainstay of pretreatment staging, radiotherapy planning, response assessment and surveillance imaging.
- MDCT has a limited role in the assessment of T1 and T2 tumours.
- EUS is considered the most accurate modality for diagnosis and assessing the depth of tumour invasion.
- Reformatted CT images in axial, coronal and sagittal planes can aid surgical planning in the patients selected for curative resection.
- Lymph node involvement is a predictor of survival.
- The commonest sites of spread are the lungs, liver, bone and adrenal glands.
- EUS is superior to CT in T staging and N staging of loco-regional disease.
- CT is useful in the assessment of distant nodal and M staging of disease.

References

1. Lee MH, Choi D, Park MJ, Lee MW. Gastric cancer: imaging and staging with MDCT based on the 7th AJCC guidelines. Abdom Imaging. 2012;37(4):531–40.
2. Kim TJ, Kim HY, Lee KW, Kim MS. Multimodality assessment of esophageal cancer: preoperative staging and monitoring of response to therapy. Radiographics. 2009;29(2):403–21.
3. Kwee RM, Kwee TC. Imaging in local staging of gastric cancer: a systematic review. J Clin Oncol. 2007;25(15):2107–16.
4. Murata Y, Suzuki S, Ohta M, Mitsunaga A, Hayashi K, Yoshida K, et al. Small ultrasonic probes for determination of the depth of superficial esophageal cancer. Gastrointest Endosc. 1996;44(1):23–8.
5. Lightdale CJ, Kulkarni KG. Role of endoscopic ultrasonography in the staging and follow-up of esophageal cancer. J Clin Oncol. 2005;23(20):4483–9.
6. Godoy MC, Bruzzi JF, Viswanathan C, Truong MT, Guimaraes MD, Hofstetter WL, et al. Multimodality imaging evaluation of esophageal cancer: staging, therapy assessment, and complications. Abdom Imaging. 2013;38(5):974–93.
7. Desai RK, Tagliabue JR, Wegryn SA, Einstein DM. CT evaluation of wall thickening in the alimentary tract. Radiographics. 1991;11(5):771–83. discussion 84.
8. Casson AG, Darnton SJ, Subramanian S, Hiller L. What is the optimal distal resection margin for esophageal carcinoma? Ann Thorac Surg. 2000;69(1):205–9.
9. Catalano MF, Sivak Jr MV, Rice T, Gragg LA, Van Dam J. Endosonographic features predictive of lymph node metastasis. Gastrointest Endosc. 1994;40(4):442–6.
10. Cerfolio RJ, Bryant AS, Ohja B, Bartolucci AA, Eloubeidi MA. The accuracy of endoscopic ultrasonography with fine-needle aspiration, integrated positron emission tomography with

computed tomography, and computed tomography in restaging patients with esophageal cancer after neoadjuvant chemoradiotherapy. J Thorac Cardiovasc Surg. 2005;129(6): 1232–41.

11. Westerterp M, van Westreenen HL, Reitsma JB, Hoekstra OS, Stoker J, Fockens P, et al. Esophageal cancer: CT, endoscopic US, and FDG PET for assessment of response to neoadjuvant therapy--systematic review. Radiology. 2005;236(3):841–51.

Basic Principles of PET-CT Imaging

5

Deborah Tout, John Dickson, and Andy Bradley

Contents

5.1 Introduction

PET-CT imaging has become a very powerful tool in cancer imaging; it utilises the detection of the radiation emitted from radionuclides that decay by positron (β^+) emission. This chapter looks into the physical principles of this technique, factors that affect the quality of the images produced and some of the artefacts and problems that may be encountered.

D. Tout (✉)
Biomedical Technology Services, Gold Coast University Hospital,
Southport, QLD, Australia
e-mail: Deborah.Tout@health.qld.gov.uk

J. Dickson
Department of Nuclear Medicine, University College London Hospitals
NHS Foundation Trust, London, UK

A. Bradley
Nuclear Medicine Centre, Manchester Royal Infirmary, Manchester, UK
e-mail: Andy.Bradley@cmft.nhs.uk

© Springer International Publishing Switzerland 2016
T.A. Szyszko (ed.), *PET/CT in Oesophageal and Gastric Cancer*, Clinicians' Guides
to Radionuclide Hybrid Imaging, DOI 10.1007/978-3-319-29240-3_5

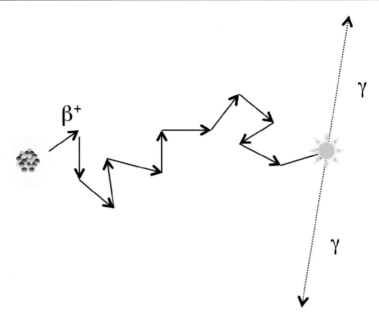

Fig. 5.1 During a nuclear decay, a positron is emitted from a nucleus and undergoes a series of interactions with atoms in the surrounding tissue. When its kinetic energy is almost zero, it and a neighbouring electron annihilate turning the mass of the two particles into energy in the form of two 511 keV photons. (Nucleus and random walk are not to scale)

5.2   Positron Emission Tomography (PET)

Positron emission tomography (PET) is the imaging of radiopharmaceuticals labelled with positron-emitting radionuclides. Positrons are the positively charged antimatter version of the electron and are ejected during the radioactive decay of a proton-rich nucleus; during this decay process, a proton in the nucleus is converted into a neutron. The positron is ejected from the nucleus carrying a lot of kinetic energy; it then travels a short distance and undergoes a number of interactions with the surrounding atoms. In each interaction, the positron loses some kinetic energy and changes its direction of travel, following a random path through the surrounding matter. When the positron is at rest, it annihilates with a nearby electron. Due to the conservation of energy, the energy associated with their combined mass (rest mass energy; $E = mc^2$) is converted to two annihilation photons each with energy of 511 keV. Conservation of momentum dictates that the two photons are emitted from the point of annihilation travelling in opposite directions (Fig. 5.1). These properties, the instantaneous production of two photons of equal energy travelling 180 degrees to each other, are the basis of the PET imaging technique used to localise where the original annihilation event occured within the patient.

A PET scanner is composed of several rings of small crystal scintillation detectors. Each detector is a few millimetres in size, and a group of them are formed

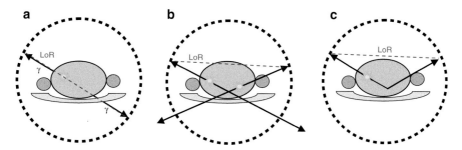

Fig. 5.2 Coincidence events in PET. (**a**) A true event with correct line of response (*LoR*), (**b**) a random event with two unrelated annihilations registering an incorrect line of response, (**c**) a scattered event where one photon has been scattered leading to an incorrectly positioned line of response

into a block that is typically connected to a group of four photomultiplier tubes. The scintillator detectors convert incoming photons into light before amplifying the signal using the photomultiplier tubes. When there is a positron emission within the ring of detectors, the two 511 keV photons, travelling at the speed of light, will be detected almost instantaneously (within approximately 10 ns). Photons arriving at different detectors within this coincidence timing window are called coincidence events. The line between the two detectors that detected each coincidence event is called the 'line of response'. Typically data are collected over several minutes and all detected coincidence events are grouped into parallel lines of response to form projections through the patient that are used for image reconstruction, typically using iterative reconstruction techniques. The great advantage of this type of localisation is that, unlike a gamma camera, it does not require collimators to provide positional information and therefore offers much higher sensitivity than single-photon emission tomography (SPECT).

The type of coincidence event described above is called a 'true' coincidence, and it is these signals that create the useful image. There are, however, other unwanted coincidence events that can occur (Fig. 5.2). A 'random' coincidence event is where multiple positron emissions and annihilations occurring in quick succession lead to a number of photons arriving at the detectors within the coincidence time window. If the wrong pair of detected photons is seen as the coincidence event, this will lead to an incorrect line of response. This process is called a random event as the line of response is not associated with a true annihilation event. The proportion of random events to total coincidence events increases significantly with higher activity concentrations and larger coincidence acceptance time windows, e.g., by moving from 10 to 15 ns. A 'scattered' event is where one or both photons coming from a positron-electron annihilation are scattered during their path to the detectors; the line of response will again be incorrect. The fraction of coincidence events that can be attributed to scatter increases with increased scattering material i.e. larger or denser tissue. Although unwanted coincidences can degrade image quality, all modern image reconstruction techniques use correction algorithms, which limit the effect of these types of event.

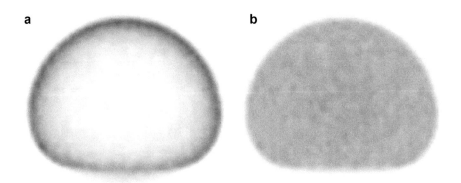

Fig. 5.3 Images of a transaxial slice through a phantom filled with a uniform solution of fluorine-18 (**a**) without correction for photon attenuation and (**b**) with attenuation correction

Along with adjustments for scattered and random events, there are other corrections that need to be applied during the reconstruction process to increase the accuracy of the final image. These include dead time corrections to deal with the high count rates found in PET, and a normalisation correction to correct for the difference in measured signal across pairs of detectors used to give the lines of response. However, the most dramatic of the corrections applied in PET is to correct for photon attenuation within the patient. Although the photons in PET are more energetic than those in single-photon tomography, both photons need to be detected for a signal to be registered; this means that the full thickness of patient tissue traversed by both photons affects the relative attenuation of signal from different parts of the patient. The effects of photon attenuation are therefore more dramatic in PET than in SPECT and lead to the classic 'hot' skin and lungs on uncorrected images (Fig. 5.3).

Exact attenuation correction (AC) is relatively straightforward so long as an accurate attenuation map is known. With the advent of PET-CT, the CT scan, which effectively is a map of attenuation at x-ray energies, can, with appropriate conversion factors, provide attenuation correction maps in a matter of seconds. The CT is mounted in the same gantry as the PET, and the bed moves the patient between the two scanners for sequential imaging. There are issues to be considered when using attenuation maps derived from CT, such as the accurate translation of attenuation coefficients from lower energy x-ray photons to 511 keV, the potential misregistration due to patient and respiratory motion, the use of contrast agents leading to incorrect attenuation maps owing to their enhanced attenuation only at the lower x-ray energies, the presence of metal artefacts and the additional radiation dose to the patient. Despite these limitations, the use of CT for AC has grown rapidly because of the low statistical noise in the attenuation maps and the addition of registered anatomical information; the fusion of CT with PET greatly enhances the interpretation of the functional information as will be seen through most of this book.

More recent technical advances include resolution (point-spread-function) modelling in PET image reconstruction resulting in significant improvements in image resolution and contrast. Also modern fast crystal detectors are able to more precisely record the difference in the arrival times of the coincidence photons, known as time-of-flight (TOF) imaging. TOF helps localise the point of origin of the annihilation event along the line of response. The reduction in noise offered by TOF can be equated to a gain in sensitivity.

An advantage of applying a comprehensive set of corrections in PET-CT is that, with the inclusion of a sensitivity calibration, there is the possibility to calculate voxel values in terms of activity concentration per unit volume (kBq/ml). This activity concentration will change with patient size or administered activity, so it becomes more useful if this uptake is represented as a value normalised by the available activity concentration in the body. This is achieved by normalising injected activity and body size (weight or lean body mass), and this leads to the semi-quantitative index known as standardised uptake value (SUV). The SUV in each voxel will equal 1 for a uniform distribution. SUV is defined as

$$SUV(g/ml) = \frac{activity\,concentration\,(kBq/ml)}{administered\,activity\,(MBq) \Big/ weight\,(kg)}.$$

SUV was defined for use in PET whole-body oncology imaging with fluorine-18-fluorodeoxyglucose (usually abbreviated as [18F]FDG or just FDG). Most PET display workstations will display PET images in SUV. Although the use of SUV is widespread, there are many factors that can affect its accuracy. It requires accurate measurement of administered activity, injection time, scan time and patient weight, and is affected by the performance characteristics of the PET scanner and image reconstruction factors. SUV also has a strong positive correlation with body weight. Heavy patients have a higher percentage of body fat that contributes to body weight but accumulates little FDG in the fasting state, so standardised uptake values (SUVs) in nonfatty tissues are increased in larger patients. SUV normalised to lean body mass or body surface area have been shown to have a lesser dependence on body weight, although SUV normalised to body weight is still the most clinically used parameter. Many physiological factors can affect SUV, including scan delay time (accumulation of FDG continues to increase over time), patient resting state, temperature, blood glucose level, insulin levels and renal clearance. In addition, FDG is not a specific tumour marker, and uptake will be high in areas affected by infective or inflammatory processes that are often seen immediately post-chemotherapy.

Several values of SUV can be quoted; the most common being SUV_{max} which is robust and relatively independent of the observer, but as it refers to a single voxel value, it is strongly affected by image noise and can change significantly depending on count statistics and reconstruction parameters. It may also not be representative of the overall uptake in a heterogeneous tumour. SUV_{mean} is more representative of the average tumour uptake and is less affected by image noise but can be prone to observer variability if freely drawn regions are used. Although the SUV formula has been criticised, the simplicity of the calculation makes it extremely attractive for routine clinical use.

Table 5.1 Properties of some radionuclides used in clinical PET imaging [1], [2]

Radionuclide	Half-life (min)	Average range (mm)	Positron fraction	Generator produced
Carbon-11	20.4	1.1	100	No
Nitrogen-13	9.96	1.5	100	No
Oxygen-15	2.03	2.5	100	No
Fluorine-18	110	0.6	97	No
Copper-64	762	0.6	18	No
Gallium-68	68	2.9	88	Yes
Rubidium-82	1.25	5.9	95	Yes

There is a wide range of positron-emitting radionuclides used in PET (Table 5.1). Many have a short half-life, which requires an expensive cyclotron production facility on the same site as the PET-CT scanner. Fluorine-18 has a slightly longer half-life, allowing it to be transported from the production facility to other imaging sites. This explains the popularity of fluorinated PET radiopharmaceuticals such as FDG. There are also longer half-life radionuclides such as copper-64 which allows imaging of pharmaceuticals with slower uptake kinetics. However, not all PET radionuclides require a cyclotron. Generators also exist, similar to the molydenum-99/technetium-99 m generator, which can produce PET radionuclides repeatedly on site. Gallium-68 and rubidium-82 are popular, short-lived, generator-produced PET radionuclides; gallium-68 comes from germanium-68 parent and rubidium-82 from strontium-82 parent.

Not all radioactive decays result in the emission of a positron; for example, with copper-64, only 18 % of decays produce positrons. This means that the sensitivity of the PET scanner to copper-64-labelled compounds is less than a fifth of that possible with fluorine-18. There may also be additional radiations resulting from the other decay routes or contaminants which can affect patient and staff radiation exposure and image quality.

The average range of the positron is important as it determines the distance the positron travels before the creation of the annihilation photons; this range is dependent on the initial energy of the positron following the radioactive decay. Because the positron moves through tissue in a random path, it is not possible to know the exact point in the tissue where the original decay took place. Spatial resolution in the images depends, to some extent, on the average range of the positron in that tissue. As a result, the spatial resolution of gallium-68 and rubidium-82 imaging will be worse than that from fluorine-18 tracers. The average positron ranges given in Table 5.1 are for soft tissue; the range of a positron will be much greater in air.

By far the most common radiopharmaceutical currently used in PET imaging is [F-18]FDG. Although FDG is a glucose analogue, it does not enter the glycolytic pathway after phosphorylation, but becomes trapped in the cell, allowing imaging of FDG concentration, which infers glycolytic rate. Both glucose and FDG are filtered by the glomeruli, but unlike glucose, FDG is not reabsorbed by the tubuli and therefore appears in urine. [F-18]FDG PET has become an important tool in oncology imaging for diagnosis and staging and to evaluate metabolic changes in tumours at the cellular level. Although very sensitive for imaging many cancer types, it is also nonspecific, detecting many other physiological processes such as inflammation and infection.

5.3   PET Scanning

PET-CT imaging usually starts with a localising scan projection radiograph often known as a 'scout' or 'topogram' where the extent of PET scanning is defined. The patient then has a CT scan of this defined length that will be used for attenuation correction and possibly uptake localisation, before moving through the scanner bore for the PET scan. The axial PET field of view which defines the amount of body that can be scanned in one stop is normally around 15 cm, although systems are now available that scan 22 cm, or even 26 cm. For brain scanning or cardiac scanning, only one field of view is required; however, in oncology imaging where the extent of disease is often of interest, whole-body imaging can be performed. This is typically done by acquiring several fields of view with a slight overlap to allow for the detector sensitivity losses at the edges of the field of view (Fig. 5.4). Each of these

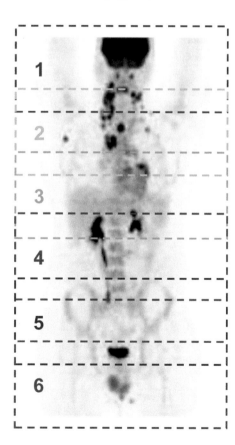

Fig. 5.4 A whole-body image is made up of multiple bed positions that are stitched together; in this example, six acquisitions are required to cover the desired length of the patient

fields of view are called a bed position, and the time of each scan at these bed positions can be between 1.5 and 5 min in duration, depending on the affinity of the radiopharmaceutical and the sensitivity of the scanner. Patients should be made comfortable and immobilised when necessary to keep the patient in the same position to maintain registration between the PET and the CT used for attenuation correction and localisation and limit movement artefacts.

For some applications, dynamic PET imaging over a single bed position can be useful to understand patient physiology. However, it is more typical to start PET imaging after a fixed period of time; this uptake or resting time is determined by the physiological uptake and excretion of the administered tracer with the aim to scan at the optimum time to have a good uptake in the target tissue with a low background circulation of the tracer in the rest of the body. For repeat imaging to assess disease progression, it is important to keep this uptake time duration similar for successive imaging, typically within +/− 5 min.

5.4   Imaging with [Fluorine-18]FDG PET

The patient must arrive well hydrated and have fasted for between 4 and 6 h to ensure blood glucose levels are low prior to injection with FDG. This is to ensure that there is limited competition between FDG and existing blood glucose, so that uptake of FDG is maximised in order to give the best possible image quality. Care needs to be taken with diabetic patients. A patient history should be taken to determine when the patient last had radiotherapy or chemotherapy. FDG uptake can be elevated as a reactive response to these treatments. It is also important to remember that FDG can be sensitive to inflammation/infection, so a general understanding of the patients' wellbeing and history of recent physical trauma (including biopsy) is necessary. For SUV calculations, patients' weight (and height if correcting for lean body mass) should be taken with reliable calibrated instruments to ensure accurate quantification of uptake. Injection of FDG should be intravenous through an indwelling cannula and the clocks used to record the injection and scan times should be calibrated; any discrepancies in the recorded times can lead to errors in the decay correction used for quantification of the uptake. All PET tracers are beta emitters (a beta particle is a high energy electron or positron), so particular care should be taken to reduce the likelihood of extravasation and local radiation burden. To assist in the quantification of FDG uptake, the exact injected activity of FDG should be recorded.

Imaging typically starts at 60 min post injection, and the patients must rest and be kept warm during this uptake period to avoid unwanted muscle or brown fat uptake. Patients are asked to void prior to imaging to reduce the activity in the bladder; full bladders containing high activity of FDG can cause difficulties in interpreting the images around this region and also increases the radiation dose to staff while the patient is positioned on the scanner bed. A multiple bed-position whole-body scan is normally performed from mid-thigh up to the base of the brain. FDG is processed via renal excretion, so it is important where possible to scan in this direction to avoid scanning a bladder that has refilled with FDG during the scan. With the patient lying supine, whole-body imaging is performed with the arms raised above the patient's head to avoid CT beam hardening artefacts and to ensure that the patient's body fits within the transaxial field of view. If head and neck imaging is required, an additional arms down scan over the head and neck area can be helpful to reduce attenuation in this area.

5.5   Artefacts

There are several artefacts that can occur in PET imaging even when all reasonable precautions are taken. One of the hardest artefacts to control is due to respiratory motion that can occur if the patient takes a large breath hold prior to or during the CT. As can be seen in Fig. 5.5(a), the result can be a banana-shaped artefact caused by mismatch of PET and CT used for attenuation correction at the base of the lung and dome of the liver. The easiest way to avoid these artefacts is to ensure that the patient is relaxed prior to imaging and asking them not to take any large intakes of breath – particularly during the CT. Other motion-related artefacts are standard patient movement such as that seen in Fig. 5.5(b). Relatively common in head and neck imaging, the mismatch of CT and PET can lead to incorrect attenuation correction and difficulty in localising features. Making the patient feel relaxed, helping

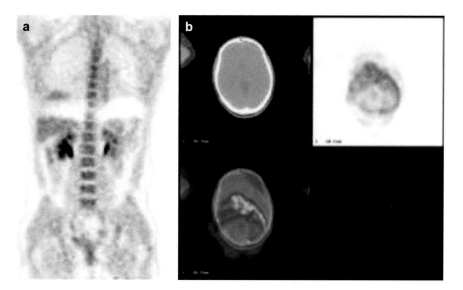

Fig. 5.5 (a) Respiratory motion artefact seen at the dome of the liver caused by mismatch of PET and CT for attenuation correction. (b) Patient motion between CT for attenuation correction and PET leading to poor correction for attenuation and localisation of tracer uptake

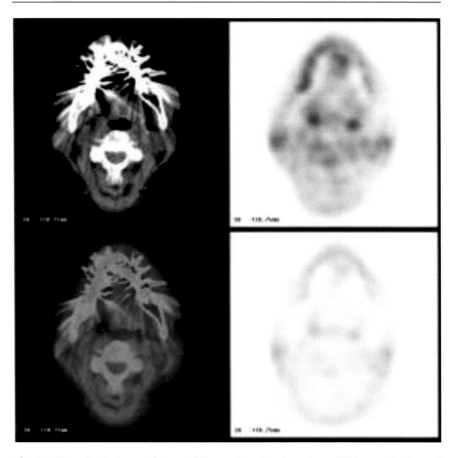

Fig. 5.6 Beam hardening artefacts on CT caused by dental amalgam. PET quantification and localisation can be difficult although non-attenuation corrected data (*bottom right panel*), may help with identifying artefacts in the attenuation corrected images (*top right panel*)

them understand the need to remain still and appropriate immobilisation can help reduce the likelihood of these artefacts.

An artefact that cannot be easily controlled is the CT x-ray beam hardening, and subsequent streaking aretefacts in the CT image, produced by metal prosthesis typically in the hip, or where the patient has metal dental work (Fig. 5.6). Many modern systems have algorithms that can help minimise these effects. Nevertheless, care must be taken when quantifying uptake in affected areas because inaccuracies in the attenuation map derived from the CT data can lead to inaccuracies in PET quantification. Another area where attenuation correction can fail is when CT contrast has been used. The conversion of the attenuation map derived from CT x-ray energies to attenuation values at PET photon energies can fail in areas of CT contrast accumulation. This is due to the elevated attenuation of contrast media, such as iodine and barium, at the lower x-ray energies due to the k-edge absorption peak; this peak does not affect the absorption of the 511 keV PET photons. As the reconstruction algorithm cannot distinguish between tissue that has a high density and less dense tissue containing CT contrast, the attenuation correction over corrects areas containing contrast. This again can lead to errors in PET quantification. If quantification is particularly important, e.g., in a trial setting, the contrast CT should be performed last after the PET data is acquired, and the attenuation correction should be performed using a low-dose CT acquired before the contrast administration.

An important tool to identiy many artefacts introduced during the attenuation correction process is the reading of PET images without attenuation correction. Although these images are then not quantitative, they can be useful to highlight areas of artefact and to assess disease within the patient.

Careful consideration of radiation protection is important due to the high-energy annihilation photons. Over ten times the thickness of lead is required to shield PET photons compared to 140 keV photons, and, immediately post injection, the dose rate from a patient administered with fluorine-18 is ten times that of a patient administered with the same activity of technetium-99 m. Extremity dose to staff can be high when handling PET tracers due to the positron radiations.

The short physical half-lives of PET tracers result in a lower patient dose than might be expected. A typical administered activity of 350 MBq [F-18]FDG corresponds to an effective dose of approximately 7 mSv, and with ongoing improvements in PET detector technology and reconstruction methods, both imaging times and typical administered activities are decreasing. The required level of CT image quality (and therefore effective dose) depends on the use of the CT data. When the CT data are used solely for AC, patient doses can be extremely low (<1 mSv). A notable improvement in image quality (and dose increase) is required if the CT data are to be used for AC and anatomical localization (typically 3–8 mSv), and a further increase in both image quality and dose is required if the CT images are to be used for diagnostic purposes, usually with the addition of contrast agents (typically >15 mSv).

Key Points
- Positron emission tomography (PET) is the imaging of radiopharmaceuticals labelled with positron-emitting radionuclides.
- Positron decay leads to two 511 keV photons following annihilation of the emitted positron and a nearby electron.
- $E = mc^2$. Positron mass $= 9.109 \times 10^{-31}$ g, speed of light $= 2.9979 \times 10^8$ m/s, $1\ eV = 1.6 \times 10^{-19}$ J. You know you want to do the calculation.
- A PET scanner is composed of several rings of scintillation detectors.
- Coincident detection of the two photons in different detectors allows an image to be formed from information gleaned by tracking 'lines of response' between these detectors.
- TOF helps localise the point of origin of the annihilation event along the line of response. This helps to decrease noise, and thereby improve signal to noise ratio.

- The sensitivity of the scanner drops towards the edges of the axial field of view of the detectors. Adjacent bed positions need to be overlapped to account for this.
- A semi-quantitative index, the standardised uptake value (SUV) is commonly used in clinical PET.
- Several values of SUV can be quoted; the most common being SUV_{max} which is relatively robust, as it is less affected by the observer than SUV_{mean}, but it is strongly affected by image noise.
- SUV_{mean} is more representative of the average tumour uptake and is less affected by image noise but can be prone to observer variability.
- To assist in the quantification of FDG uptake, the exact injected activity of FDG should be recorded.
- For SUV calculations, patients' weight (and height if correcting by lean body mass) should be taken with reliable calibrated instruments to ensure accurate quantification of uptake.
- SUVs are affected by changes in reconstruction techniques and can vary between scanners; it is only semi-quantitative.
- Careful patient preparation is important to obtain good-quality PET images.
- All PET tracers are beta emitters, so particular care should be taken to reduce the likelihood of extravasation and local radiation burden.
- There are several artefacts that can occur in PET imaging even when all reasonable precautions are taken; knowledge of these is important when interpreting images.
- The effects of photon attenuation are more dramatic in PET, and attenuation correction is essential.
- A typical administered activity of 350 MBq F-18 FDG corresponds to an effective dose of approximately 7 mSv.
- Radiation doses to staff are much higher when exposed to PET tracers than from similar activities of other technetium-based nuclear medicine tracers.

References

1. NUDAT 2.6, National Nuclear Data Centre. Brookhaven National Laboratory. http://www.nndc.bnl.gov/nudat2/.
2. Cal-Gonzalez J, et al. Positron range effects in high resolution 3D PET imaging, Nuclear Science Symposium conference record (NSS/MIC). 2009 IEEE Orlando, FL.

^{18}F-FDG and Non-FDG PET Radiopharmaceuticals

6

James Ballinger and Gopinath Gnanasegaran

Contents

6.1   Introduction

Positron emission tomography/computed tomography (PET/CT) is one of the key imaging techniques in oncology. Hybrid PET/CT provides both structural and metabolic information and in general improves sensitivity, specificity, and reporter confidence.

Fluorine-18 (^{18}F) is the most commonly used PET-emitting radionuclide label in clinical practice. It is produced using a cyclotron and has a physical half-life of 110 min. The most widely used tracer at present is the glucose analogue, 2-fluoro-2-deoxyglucose (FDG) (Table 6.1).

J. Ballinger (✉)
Division of Imaging Sciences, King's College London, London, UK
e-mail: Jim.ballinger@kcl.ac.uk

G. Gnanasegaran
Department of Nuclear Medicine, Royal Free London NHS Foundation Trust, London, UK

© Springer International Publishing Switzerland 2016
T.A. Szyszko (ed.), *PET/CT in Oesophageal and Gastric Cancer*, Clinicians' Guides
to Radionuclide Hybrid Imaging, DOI 10.1007/978-3-319-29240-3_6

43

Table 6.1 Oncology PET radiopharmaceuticals [1–11]

Class	Radiopharmaceutical	Clinical application
Oncology: 18F	Fludeoxyglucose (FDG)	Glucose metabolism
	Fluoride	Bone metabolism
	Fluoro-L-thymidine (FLT)	DNA synthesis
	Fluoromethylcholine (FCh)	Phospholipid synthesis
	Fluoroethylcholine (FEC)	Phospholipid synthesis
	Fluoroethyltyrosine (FET)	Protein synthesis
	Fluoromisonidazole (FMISO)	Hypoxia
	Fluoroazomycin arabinoside (FAZA)	Hypoxia
	Fluoroerythronitroimidazole (FETNIM)	Hypoxia
	Fluciclatide	Angiogenesis
	F-galacto-RGD	Angiogenesis
	Fluciclovine (FACBC)	Amino acid transport
	ICMT11	Apoptosis
Oncology: ^{11}C	Acetate	Membrane synthesis
	Choline	Phospholipid synthesis
	Methionine	Protein synthesis
Oncology: ^{68}Ga	DOTATOC	Somatostatin receptor
	DOTATATE	Somatostatin receptor
	HA-DOTATATE	Somatostatin receptor
	DOTANOC	Somatostatin receptor
	Somatoscan	Somatostatin receptor
	PSMA	Prostate-specific membrane antigen
	NOTA-RGD	Angiogenesis
Oncology: ^{124}I	Iodide	Sodium iodide symporter
	MIBG	Neuronal activity

6.2 PET Radiopharmaceuticals

6.2.1 ^{18}F-FDG

^{18}F-FDG has a role in localising, characterising, staging and monitoring treatment response and evaluating recurrent disease in a variety of cancer types. However, increased FDG uptake is not specific to cancer cells. FDG accumulates in cells, in proportion to glucose utilisation [1–5]. In general, increased glucose uptake is a characteristic of most cancers and is in part mediated by overexpression of the GLUT-1 glucose transporter and increased hexokinase activity [1–5]. The net result is an increased accumulation of FDG within tumour cells at a rate greater than in normal tissue. Active inflammatory changes can also result in increased FDG uptake, due to increased glucose utilisation by activated granulocytes and mononuclear cells [1–5] (Tables 6.1, 6.2, and 6.3). The principal route of excretion of FDG from the bloodstream is via the urinary tract. The biodistribution of ^{18}F-FDG varies on several factors such as (a) fasting state, (b) medications, (c) duration of the

Table 6.2   Properties of positron-emitting radionuclides used in clinical practice

Radionuclide	Half-life	Positron energy (max, MeV)	Other emissions	Means of production
Carbon-11	20 min	0.96	–	Cyclotron
Nitrogen-13	10 min	1.20	–	Cyclotron
Oxygen-15	2 min	1.74	–	Cyclotron
Fluorine-18	110 min	0.63	–	Cyclotron
Copper-62	10 min	2.93	–	Generator
Copper-64	13 h	0.65	Beta, gamma	Cyclotron
Gallium-68	68 min	1.83	–	Generator
Rubidium-82	76 s	3.15	–	Generator
Zirconium-89	79 h	0.40	Gamma	Cyclotron
Iodine-124	4.2 days	1.50	Gamma	Cyclotron

Table 6.3   Common radiopharmaceuticals and their mechanism of uptake [11]

Radiotracer	Mechanism of uptake
^{18}F-Fluorodeoxyglucose (FDG)	Uptake by GLUT-1 transporter followed by phosphorylation by hexokinase
Sodium ^{18}F-fluoride (NaF)	Incorporated within hydroxyapatite in proportion to bone metabolism
^{68}Ga-labelled peptides	Binds to peptide receptor, most commonly somatostatin receptor
^{18}F-Choline (FCh) ^{11}C-Choline	Incorporation into phosphatidylcholine as part of cell wall synthesis
^{11}C-Methionine	Amino acid transport
^{18}F-Fluorothymidine (FLT) ^{11}C-Thymidine	Phosphorylated by thymidine kinase in proliferating cells; FLT not incorporated into DNA
^{82}Rb-Chloride	Transported into myocardial cells by sodium-potassium ATPase in proportion to regional myocardial perfusion

uptake period post tracer injection, (d) variant metabolism and (e) incidental pathology and is discussed in detail in Chap. 8.

6.2.2   Non-FDG Radiopharmaceuticals

In addition to ^{18}F-FDG, there are several cyclotron- and generator-based radiolabelled molecules used in clinical PET/CT imaging. Sodium fluoride (^{18}F-NaF), ^{68}Ga-labelled peptides, ^{18}F-choline, ^{11}C-choline, etc., each have clinical applications and are discussed in detail in this pocket book series titled *PET Radiotracers*. While FDG is the workhorse of oncological PET imaging, it is nonspecific as it monitors the ubiquitous process of glucose metabolism. Alternative tracers tend to be more specific in their targeting and application. Some attempt to probe the hallmarks of cancer, such as uncontrolled proliferation, angiogenesis, evasion of apoptosis, and tissue invasion. Tumour microenvironment, such as hypoxia, has also been probed. However, the tracers which have come into wider use tend to be those which monitor specific features such as membrane synthesis incorporating choline, prostate-specific membrane antigen (PSMA) expression, and somatostatin receptor expression.

Conclusion
It is likely that the range of positron-emitting radiopharmaceuticals in routine clinical use will continue to expand in the coming years.

Key Points
Fluorine-18 (^{18}F) is the most commonly used PET-emitting radionuclide label in clinical practice.

Fluorine-18 (^{18}F) is produced using a cyclotron and has a physical half-life of 110 min.

The most widely used tracer at present is the glucose analogue, 2-fluoro-2-deoxyglucose (FDG). FDG is the workhorse of oncological PET imaging.

FDG is actively transported into the cell mediated by a group of structurally related glucose transport proteins (GLUT).

Increased FDG uptake is not specific to cancer cells and often will accumulate in areas with increased metabolism and glycolysis.

The principal route of excretion of FDG from the bloodstream is via the urinary tract.

Non-FDG tracers include sodium fluoride (^{18}F-NaF), ^{68}Ga-labelled peptides, ^{18}F-choline, and ^{11}C-choline.

References

1. Torizuka T, Tamaki N, Inokuma T, et al. In vivo assessment of glucose metabolism in hepatocellular carcinoma with FDG-PET. J Nucl Med. 1995;36:1811–7.
2. Cook GJR, Fogelman I, Maisey MN. Normal physiological and benign pathological variants of ^{18}F-FDG PET scanning: potential for error in interpretation. Semin Nucl Med. 1996;26:308–14.
3. Warburg O. On the origin of cancer cells. Science. 1956;123:309–14.
4. Cook GJR, Maisey MN, Fogelman I. Normal variants, artefacts and interpretative pitfalls in PET imaging with ^{18}F-fluoro-2-deoxyglucose and carbon-11-methionine. Eur J Nucl Med. 1999;26:1363–78.
5. Culverwell AD, Scarsbrook AF, Chowdhury FU. False-positive uptake on 2-[^{18}F]-fluoro-2-deoxy-D-glucose (FDG) positron-emission tomography/computed tomography (PET/CT) in oncological imaging. Clin Radiol. 2011;66:366–82.
6. Shreve PD, Anzai Y, Wahl RL. Pitfalls in oncologic diagnosis with FDG PET imaging: physiologic and benign variants. Radiographics. 1999;19:61–77.
7. Delbeke D, Coleman RE, Guiberteau MJ, et al. Procedure guideline for tumour imaging with ^{18}F-FDG PET/CT 1.0. J Nucl Med. 2006;47:885–95.
8. Boellaard R, O'Doherty MJ, Weber WA, et al. FDG PET and PET/CT: EANM procedure guidelines for tumour PET imaging: version 1.0. Eur J Nucl Med Mol Imaging. 2010;37:181–200.

9. Segall G, Delbeke D, Stabin MG, et al. SNM practice guideline for sodium 18F-fluoride PET/CT bone scans 1.0. J Nucl Med. 2010;51:1813–20.
10. Virgolini I, Ambrosini V, Bomanji JB, et al. Procedure guidelines for PET/CT tumour imaging with ⁶⁸Ga-DOTA-conjugated peptides: ⁶⁸Ga-DOTA-TOC, ⁶⁸Ga-DOTA-NOC, ⁶⁸Ga-DOTA-TATE. Eur J Nucl Med Mol Imaging. 2010;37:2004–10.
11. Juweid ME, Cheson BD. Positron-emission tomography and assessment of cancer therapy. N Engl J Med. 2006;2(354):496–507.

PET/CT Imaging: Patient Instructions and Preparation

7

Shaunak Navalkissoor, Thomas Wagner,
Gopinath Gnanasegaran, Teresa A. Szyszko,
and Jamshed B. Bomanji

Contents

7.1 Introduction

^{18}F-FDG PET is a frequently used imaging modality in the evaluation of cancer patients. A high-quality study performed ^{18}F-FDG PET study should be repeatable (same result produced if imaged on the same system) and reproducible (similar result if imaged at different sites). An essential component of this is adequate patient preparation to ensure study reproducibility and technical quality. Rigorous instructions should be followed regarding patient procedure. In addition, adequate referral information is important so that the correct timing of study and imaging protocol can be followed, e.g. lung gating for a base of lung lesion. This section addresses

S. Navalkissoor (✉) • T. Wagner • G. Gnanasegaran
Department of Nuclear Medicine, Royal Free London NHS Foundation Trust, London, UK
e-mail: s.navalkissoor@nhs.net

T.A. Szyszko
King's College and Guy's and St Thomas' PET Centre, Division of Imaging Sciences and Biomedical Engineering, Kings College London, St Thomas' Hospital, London, UK

J.B. Bomanji
Department of Nuclear Medicine, University College London Hospitals NHS Foundation Trust, London, UK

© Springer International Publishing Switzerland 2016
T.A. Szyszko (ed.), *PET/CT in Oesophageal and Gastric Cancer*, Clinicians' Guides to Radionuclide Hybrid Imaging, DOI 10.1007/978-3-319-29240-3_7

Table 7.1 Contents of PET/CT request [1–5]

1. Patient name, date of birth, address and hospital identifier number
2. Clinical indication
3. Clinical question to be answered
4. Oncological history: site of tumour (if known), recent biopsy (site, date of biopsy and results if known) and comorbidity
5. Drug allergies and allergy to contrast agents
6. Diabetes status, if relevant (IDDM, NIDDM), and treatment
7. Renal function
8. Therapeutic interventions: type and date of last treatment (chemotherapy, surgery, radiotherapy, bone marrow stimulants and steroids administration)
9. Result and availability of previous imaging
10. Height and body weight
11. Referring clinician's contact details: (a) to discuss about the referral, (b) to contact during emergency and (c) to send the reports
12. Date at which results of the PET or PET/CT study must be available

some of these issues, and summaries of required clinical information, patient preparation, procedure and imaging parameters are shown in Tables 7.1, 7.2 and 7.3.

FDG is a glucose analogue and is transferred intracellularly by glucose transporters. Many tumour cells overexpress glucose transporter proteins and hexokinase intracellularly, which allows FDG to be used to image these tumours.

7.2   Patient Preparation

One of the main aims in patient preparation is to reduce the hyperinsulinemic state, which occurs with recent glucose ingestion. Increased glucose levels cause competitive inhibition of ^{18}F-FDG uptake by the cells leading to decreased tumour (or other active process) to background ratio. Also increased insulin secondary to elevated blood glucose increases translocation of GLUT4, thereby shunting ^{18}F-FDG to organs with high density of insulin receptors (e.g. skeletal muscles). Patients should thus fast for at least 6 h prior to the study to ensure low insulin levels. Recent EANM guidelines suggest that patients with blood glucose <11 mmol/l can have FDG administered, whilst patients with glucose >11 mmol/l need to be rescheduled. Patients with diabetes (particularly with insulin-based treatments) need to be carefully scheduled to avoid a hyperinsulinemic state. (An example of scheduling includes a late morning appointment with an early breakfast and insulin injection.)

If glucose control is not achieved, then the PET scan can be rescheduled.

Other patient preparations also aim to reduce tracer uptake in normal tissues, thus increasing target and nontarget uptake. Patients should be hydrated adequately to decrease the concentration of FDG in the urine, decreasing artefacts and potentially reducing radiation dose. Drinking water is permitted; however, flavoured water contains sugar and cannot be consumed prior to the PET scan. Patients should be advised to dress warmly on the way to the PET suite and should be kept in a warm room prior to the administration of FDG. This is to avoid accumulation of

Table 7.2 General instructions for an ^{18}F-FDG PET scan [1–5]

Appointment:
1. Send leaflets related to the scan and instructions
2. Confirm appointment
3. Medications list if any
4. History of diabetes, fasting state and recent infection/intervention

Before arrival:
1. Fast, except for water (for at least 6 h before the injection of ^{18}F-FDG for most studies, at least 4 h before dedicated neuroimaging). Avoid chewing gum
   (a) Morning appointment: patient should not eat after midnight [preferably have a light meal (no alcohol) during the evening prior to the PET study]
   (b) Afternoon appointment PET study: patient may have a light breakfast before 8.00 a.m. (no sugars or sugar-containing fillings/products)
2. Advise adequate pre-hydration
3. Intravenous fluids containing dextrose or parenteral feedings should be withheld for 4–6 h before radiotracer injection
4. Consider if intravenous contrast material is to be used for CT

Before injecting:
1. The blood glucose level should be checked and documented
   FDG PET study can be performed: *if plasma glucose level is <11 mmol/l (or <200 mg/dl)*
   FDG PET study should be rescheduled: *if plasma glucose level is ≥11 mmol/l (or >200 mg/dl) depending on patients circumstances*
2. Keep the patient in a warm room for 30–60 min before the injection and during the uptake period and maintain warmth with blankets during scan to reduce uptake in the brown fat. (*Lorazepam, diazepam and beta-blockers may help to reduce uptake by brown fat uptake if problematic*)
3. Check patient's ability to lie still for the duration of the scan and ability to put his or her arms overhead
4. Ask for history of claustrophobia
5. If intravenous contrast material is to be used, patients should be screened for iodinated contrast material allergy, renal disease and use of metformin for diabetes mellitus treatment
6. Take a brief history and document site of malignancy, including recent investigations and treatment history: surgery, radiation, chemotherapy

Table 7.3 ^{18}F-FDG PET/CT imaging parameters [1–5]

Routine imaging: skull base to upper thigh

Additional views: lower limb views, dedicated head and neck or occasionally scan to vertex are acquired as necessary

Brain imaging is frequently omitted in many institutions routinely (poor sensitivity of FDG PET for brain metastases)

Typical adult administered activities: 185–370 MBq (5–10 mCi), up to 400 MBq

Largest effective dose administered: urinary bladder

Whole-body effective dose of PET study is approximately 0.02 mSv/MBq or 7–8 mSv for an adult administered activity of 370 MBq. CT dose depends on local protocol

FDG in activated brown fat. In some cases with no contraindications to oral beta-blockers, propranolol (1 mg/kg, maximum 40 mg) should be given at least 90 min before FDG injection to reduce FDG uptake in brown adipose tissue. This is especially important in young patients. Strenuous physical activity should be avoided for

Table 7.4 Example of low-carbohydrate high-fat diet provided to patients prior to FDG PET cardiac imaging

Do not eat the following:
Sugar in any form (including natural's sugars in fruits)
No starches, e.g. pasta, breads, cereals, rice and potatoes
No vegetables with high carbohydrate content, no carrots or beetroot
No chocolates, sweets, chewing gums, mints and cough syrups
No processed products, e.g. processed deli meats
No sweetener substitutes like Canderel or Splenda
No milk or milk products
No cheese or cheese products
No nuts
No fruits
No alcohol
You can eat the following:
Poultry: fatty unsweetened chicken and turkey (fried or boiled, *NOT* grilled)
Meats: fatty unsweetened, red meat, bacon, ham (fried or boiled, *NOT* T grilled)
Fish: any fish (fatty unsweetened, fried or boiled, *NOT* grilled)
Shellfish: any non-processed shellfish
Eggs: fried, scrambled preparation without milk, omelette prepared without milk or vegetables
Butter and margarine
Vegetables: cucumber, broccoli, lettuce, celery, mushroom, green pepper, cabbage, spinach, asparagus, radish
Drinks: mineral water (still or sparkling), coffee, tea, herbal tea (without milk or sugar)

at least 6 h prior to the scan to avoid excessive skeletal uptake. During the uptake period, the patient should not talk and avoid reading or chewing, to minimise uptake in these respective muscles.

If a lesion near the myocardium or the myocardium itself is being evaluated for suspected disease, careful patient preparation is required to limit cardiac uptake. A low-carbohydrate, high-fat, high-protein diet for at least 24 h before the scan (Table 7.4) and extended fasting for 18 h before the scan are recommended to switch the myocardial energy substrate from glucose to fatty acids. This is coupled with one or two intravenous bolus of heparin (50 IU/kg) given 90 min prior to[18]F-FDG injection for suppression of myocardial FDG uptake.

Review of patients' medication should be performed, e.g. steroids in high doses may cause hyperglycaemic states and, in patients with suspected vasculitis, may reduce the sensitivity of the test; metformin may cause diffuse large bowel uptake due to increased glucose utilisation of the intestinal mucosa. If intravenous contrast is going to be administered, metformin needs to be withheld on the day of the test and for a further 48 h.

7.3   Timing of FDG PET Scan After Treatment

When the PET scan is being protocolled, adequate information about previous treatments should be available to the authoriser to ensure accurate timing, e.g. in chemotherapy response assessments in lymphoma, the FDG PET scan should not be performed too early to avoid false negatives due to tumour stunning or false positives due to inflammatory uptake. An interval of at least 10 days should be allowed post chemotherapy (interim PET) or at least 3 weeks at the end of chemotherapy to allow evaluation of response to chemotherapy. If patients are undergoing radiotherapy, the recommended post-therapy interval is 2–3 months.

Key Points
- Rigorous instructions should be followed regarding patient procedure.
- Adequate referral information is important so that the correct timing of study and imaging protocol can be followed.
- Increased glucose levels cause competitive inhibition of ^{18}F-FDG uptake.
- Increased insulin secondary to elevated blood glucose increases translocation of GLUT4.
- Patients should thus fast for at least 6 h prior to the study to ensure low insulin levels.
- Patients with blood glucose <11 mmol/l can have FDG administered, whilst patients with glucose >11 mmol/l need to be rescheduled (EANM guidelines).
- Patients with diabetes (particularly with insulin-based treatments) need to be carefully scheduled to avoid a hyperinsulinemic state.
- Patients should be hydrated adequately to decrease the concentration of FDG in the urine, decreasing artefacts and potentially reducing radiation dose.
- Keep the patient in a warm room for 30–60 min before the FDG injection.
- Strenuous physical activity should be avoided for at least 6 h prior to the scan.
- An interval of at least 10 days should be allowed post chemotherapy (interim PET) or at least 3 weeks at the end of chemotherapy to allow evaluation of response to chemotherapy.
- In patients undergoing radiotherapy, the recommended post-therapy interval is 3 months.

References

1. Delbeke D, Coleman RE, Guiberteau MJ, et al. Procedure guideline for tumour imaging with ^{18}F-FDG PET/CT 1.0. J Nucl Med. 2006;47(5):885–95.
2. Boellaard R, O'Doherty MJ, Weber WA, et al. FDG PET and PET/CT: EANM procedure guidelines for tumour PET imaging: version 1.0. Eur J Nucl Med Mol Imaging. 2010;37(1):181–200.
3. Boellaard R, Delgado-Bolton R, Oyen WGJ, Giammarile F, Tatsch K, Eschner W, et al. FDG PET/CT: EANM procedure guidelines for tumour imaging: version 2.0. Eur J Nucl Med Mol Imaging. 2015;42:328–54.
4. Juweid ME, Cheson BD. Positron-emission tomography and assessment of cancer therapy. N Engl J Med. 2006;354(5):496–507.
5. Graham MM, Wahl RL, Hoffmans JM, Yaps JT, Sunderland JT, et al. Summary of the UPICT protocol for 18F-FDG PET/CT imaging in oncology clinical trials. J Nucl Med. 2015;56:955–61.

^{18}F-FDG PET/CT Imaging: Normal Variants, Pitfalls and Artefacts

8

Kanhaiyalal Agrawal, Gopinath Gnanasegaran, Evangelia Skoura, Alexis Corrigan, and Teresa A. Szyszko

Contents

8.1   Introduction

In recent years, positron emission tomography (PET)/computed tomography (CT) has gained widespread clinical acceptance in oncology. It is being used extensively in the diagnosis, staging, restaging and therapy response evaluation of tumours (Table 8.1) along with several benign indications in cardiology and neurology.

K. Agrawal (✉)
Department of Nuclear Medicine and PET/CT, North City Hospital, Kolkata, India
e-mail: drkanis@gmail.com

G. Gnanasegaran
Department of Nuclear Medicine, Royal Free London NHS Foundation Trust, London, UK

E. Skoura
Institute of Nuclear Medicine, UCLH, London, UK

A. Corrigan
Department of Nuclear Medicine and Radiology, Maidstone and Tunbridge Wells NHS Trust, Tunbridge Wells, UK

T.A. Szyszko
King's College and Guy's and St Thomas' PET Centre, Division of Imaging Sciences and Biomedical Engineering, Kings College London, St Thomas' Hospital, London, UK

© Springer International Publishing Switzerland 2016   55
T.A. Szyszko (ed.), *PET/CT in Oesophageal and Gastric Cancer*, Clinicians' Guides
to Radionuclide Hybrid Imaging, DOI 10.1007/978-3-319-29240-3_8

Table 8.1 Clinical role of PET/CT imaging in oncology

Diagnosis
Localisation
Staging
Restaging
Treatment response
Recurrent disease or relapse
Radiotherapy planning
Guiding metabolic biopsy
Grading tumours

Fluorine-18 (^{18}F) 2-fluoro-2-deoxy-D-glucose (FDG) is the most commonly used positron-emitting radiotracer in PET/CT studies. In this chapter, we will mainly focus on normal variants and artefacts in ^{18}F-FDG PET/CT studies.

^{18}F-FDG is a glucose analogue labelled with a positron-emitting isotope ^{18}F. It is transported into cells through glucose transporters and phosphorylated by enzyme hexokinase to ^{18}F-FDG-6-phosphate [1]. The cell membrane is impermeable to both glucose-6-phosphate and ^{18}F-FDG-6-phosphate. However, the latter cannot be degraded further via the glycolysis pathway and remains trapped within the cell. ^{18}F-FDG is accumulated in malignant tissues more avidly than within the normal tissues due to increased glucose metabolism rate, increased expression of glucose transporters and highly active hexokinase bound to mitochondria of malignant tissue in comparison to normal tissue. However, ^{18}F-FDG uptake is also known to occur in inflammation, infection and healing tissues. This is partly due to the fact that infiltrated granulocytes and tissue macrophages use glucose as energy source. In inflammation, the granulocytes and macrophages are activated, and hence, glucose metabolism increases [2].

There can be variable degree of physiological tracer uptake in the various organs in the ^{18}F-FDG PET/CT scans (Fig. 8.1) (Table 8.2) [3–16]. Recognition of physiological tracer distribution is essential in avoiding incorrect image interpretation. Sometimes special patient preparation is needed to suppress the physiological tracer uptake to identify pathology in some organs [14]. It is important that patient is relaxed on the day of the study and should maintain silence to avoid muscle uptake [5]. Brown fat uptake can be suppressed by keeping the patient warm or sometimes by administration of oral beta-blockers and benzodiazepines, especially in patients with suspected pathology in the neck and mediastinum. Similarly, cardiac ^{18}F-FDG PET imaging needs either prolonged fasting or special low-carbohydrate high-fat diet to suppress physiological uptake in the myocardium [14]. It is always better to avoid administering insulin to the patient on the day of study as this may lead to increased background activity in the fat and muscles and decreases uptake in the tumour [5]. Physiological tracer activity in the urinary tract may mask pathologic conditions. Good hydration and use of intravenous diuretics should be considered to decrease the urinary stasis in the kidneys and ureters. It also dilutes the urine activity in the urinary bladder and helps in better evaluation of surrounding structures like the prostate gland.

Fig. 8.1 Maximum intensity projection (MIP) ¹⁸F-FDG PET/CT image shows normal physiological tracer distribution in the brain, heart, liver, stomach, bowel and testes and excretion through kidneys into urinary bladder. [It is essential to recognise normal physiological uptake in order to interpret FDG PET images correctly]

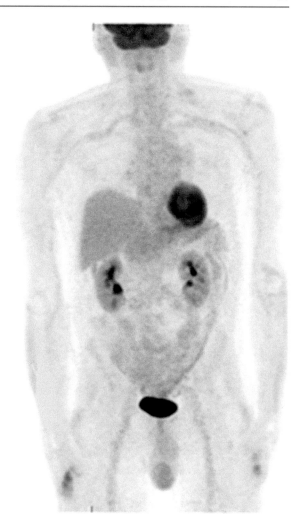

¹⁸F-FDG PET study immediately after chemotherapy and radiotherapy introduces false-positive findings [5–9, 12, 13, 16]. Hence, at least a gap of 3 weeks following chemotherapy and 3 months following radiotherapy to perform ¹⁸F-FDG PET study should be considered to reduce the false positives. Scanning performed immediately after surgery or biopsy may show falsely increased tracer localisation due to post-surgical inflammation. In addition, infection such as pneumonia, tuberculosis and osteomyelitis leads to false positives in oncology patients [2, 5–9, 12, 13, 16].

Imaging on hybrid PET/CT scanners may lead to misregistration due to differences in breathing patterns and patient movement between CT and PET image acquisitions [5–9]. Patient movement may be avoided by instructing the patient to lie down still during the scan or sometimes by using sedation judiciously in patient

Table 8.2 ^{18}F-FDG PET scan appearances and physiological variation [5–9, 12, 13, 16]

Organ	Physiological uptake/variation	Comments
Brain	Intense uptake in the cortex, basal ganglia and thalami (Fig. 8.2a)	Metastases are best assessed with MRI
Breast	Low-grade diffuse uptake within the breast is normal due to proliferative glandular tissue. Higher uptake may be seen in adolescent girls with dense breasts (Fig. 8.2d) The uptake in the areola is variable, but prominent uptake may be seen	Markedly increased in lactating breast. The amount of radioactivity within milk from breasts is low. The infant is more likely to receive radiation exposure from close contact with the breast, rather than from milk
Bone marrow	Low diffuse uptake in haematopoietic bone marrow is physiological	
Brown fat	Neck, paraspinal, retroperitoneal fat, etc.	Patient waiting areas should be kept warm. Drug intervention may be helpful
Endometrium	Central moderate uptake within the uterus is normal during ovulatory and secretory phases	Menstrual history is important and tracer uptake may be pathological in postmenopausal women
GI tract	Highly variable Increased tracer uptake with a focal, diffuse or segmental distribution could be physiologic and more marked in patients taking the antidiabetic drug such as metformin (Fig. 8.15)	Focal areas of increased uptake usually warrants further evaluation
Heart	Variable ranging from negligible to intense uptake (Fig. 8.3) depending on its metabolic state at the time of the study	Partly depends on fasting state (may be suppressed by prolonged fast or low-carbohydrate high-fat diet). However, in PET cardiac imaging, the main aim is to increase cardiac uptake of FDG, and increasing uptake in cardiac cells can be achieved by increasing the serum insulin level or decreasing the free fatty acid level
Liver	Mild to moderate uptake (relatively homogeneous) (Fig. 8.2e)	
Muscles	Mild uptake is physiological Symmetrical diaphragmatic, intercostals and strap muscle uptake could be physiological or may relate to increased respiratory effort in patients with pulmonary disease (Fig. 8.4)	Tracer uptake is increased in patients who are not adequately fasted or following exercise/exertion (thorough clinical history is useful in these cases) (Fig. 8.5)
Ovary	During mid-cycle, moderate increased uptake in the adnexae is normal (unilateral or bilateral) (Fig. 8.6)	Menstrual history is important. Tracer uptake may be pathological in postmenopausal women. Bilateral adnexal and uterine activity is likely to represent physiological ovarian and uterine uptake in a premenopausal woman

Table 8.2 (continued)

Organ	Physiological uptake/variation	Comments
Ocular muscles	Moderate or intense tracer uptake Related to eye movement during uptake period (Fig. 8.2b)	Patient should be advised to rest quietly in darkened room
Salivary glands	Low-grade tracer uptake is physiological and is often symmetrical	
Spleen	Homogeneous uptake slightly less than to liver (Fig. 8.2e)	
Testes	Mild to moderate symmetrical uptake is physiological and declines with age (Fig. 8.2h)	
Thymus	Low to moderate uptake in children and young adults is normal (Fig. 8.7)	Often reactivated post chemotherapy and tracer uptake should be correlated with age of patient and medical history/treatment
Thyroid	Diffuse or focal uptake are often seen (Fig. 8.11d)	Diffuse uptake is seen in patients with Graves' disease, subacute thyroiditis or Hashimoto's thyroiditis Focal uptake is often seen in thyroid nodules and should be further evaluated with fine needle aspiration to rule out sinister pathology
Tonsils	Common and variable. Often symmetrical and may relate to local infection/inflammation (Fig. 8.8)	
Urinary tract	Increased activity within urinary tract is normal (Fig. 8.2f)	Good hydration and voiding is advised before imaging
Vocal cords	Variable – moderate and symmetrical (Fig. 8.9)	Relates to phonation during uptake period. Unilateral uptake requires further evaluation – may relate to tumour or potentially unilateral vocal cord palsy

with severe pain and in children. Misregistration can be minimised by performing the CT scan during normal expiration. In hybrid PET/CT studies, low-dose CT data is used for attenuation correction of PET data. However, high-density contrast agents or metallic objects may lead to overcorrection if CT data is used for attenuation correction [5]. This leads to falsely increased tracer activity at these sites. Similarly, parts of the brain may show falsely decreased uptake due to under attenuation correction of PET data if there is patient movement. Reviewing the non-attenuation corrected data is helpful in avoiding such misinterpretation. Another potential problem with low-dose CT for attenuation correction is beam hardening artefacts, particularly in larger patients. This can lead to inaccurate attenuation correction. However, recently with many centres using diagnostic quality CT in PET/CT studies, this issue is not very frequent. Also, as this is commonly caused by the patient's arms being in the field of view, it can be avoided by placing arms above the head during imaging. However, if the head and neck is the area of interest, it is advised to

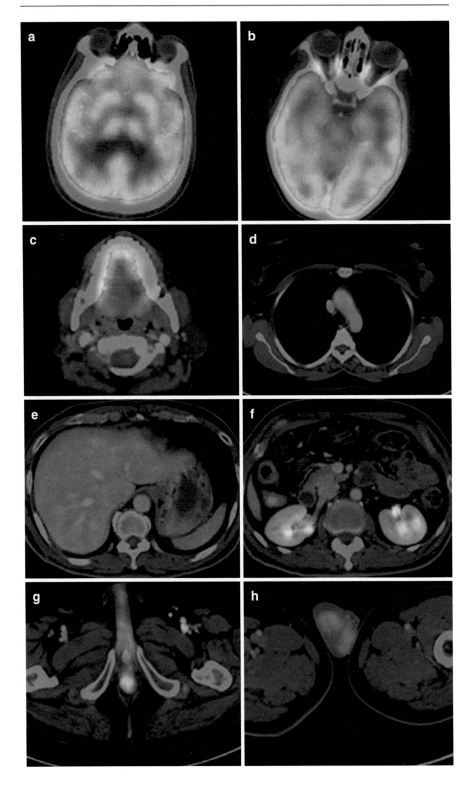

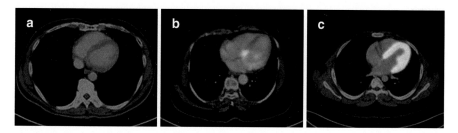

Fig. 8.3 ¹⁸F-FDG PET/CT studies show different patterns of physiological tracer uptake in the myocardium varying from negligible (**a**), segmental (**b**) to diffuse intense uptake (**c**). [Variable myocardial uptake depends partly on fasting state and may be suppressed by prolonged fast or a low-carbohydrate high-fat diet. In PET cardiac imaging, the main aim is to increase cardiac uptake of FDG by increasing the serum insulin level]

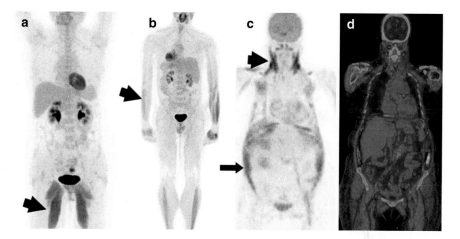

Fig. 8.4 (**a, b**) MIP ¹⁸F-FDG PET image shows uptake in the skeletal muscles (*arrows*) likely due to overuse or muscular strain. This may obscure peripheral primary tumours, e.g. in melanoma. (**c, d**) MIP and coronal fused ¹⁸F-FDG PET/CT images show increased tracer uptake in the respiratory muscles in a patient with breathing difficulty. The diffuse uptake in the abdominal muscles may mimic peritoneal uptake and caution is advised. [In general, exercising muscles, postexercise, uses glucose (energy substrate), and in contrast, resting muscles predominantly use free fatty acids. Therefore, patients should avoid strenuous/severe exercise for at least a day prior to imaging]

Fig. 8.2 Axial fused PET/CT images from different ¹⁸F-FDG PET/CT studies show physiological tracer uptake in the (**a**) brain, (**b**) medial and lateral rectus muscles of orbits, (**c**) tongue, (**d**) breasts, (**e**) liver and collapsed stomach wall, (**f**) kidneys, (**g**) rectum and (**h**) testes

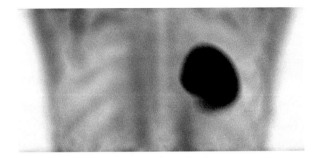

Fig. 8.5 MIP^{18}F-FDG PET image of a patient for cardiac viability study shows diffuse increased tracer uptake in the muscles due to glucose loading and insulin administration. [Diffuse muscle uptake can often be seen when the serum insulin level is elevated/increased]

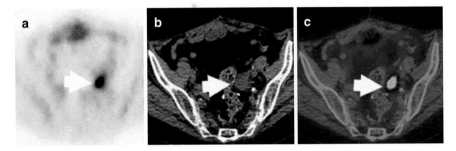

Fig. 8.6 Transaxial PET (**a**), CT (**b**) and fused (**c**) images show. Physiological tracer uptake in the left adnexa (*arrow*). [Adnexal and uterine activity is likely to represent physiological ovarian and uterine uptake in a premenopausal woman and is usually seen mid-cycle. A corpus luteum cyst can present as a "ring" for peripheral uptake in the adnexa. It is important to check the patient's menstrual history. Increased adnexal or uterine uptake in a postmenopausal woman warrants further investigation]

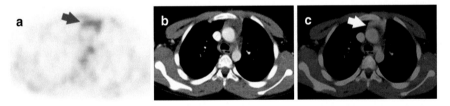

Fig. 8.7 Transaxial PET (**a**), CT (**b**) and fused (**c**) images demonstrate diffuse and homogeneous uptake (*arrow* in **a**, **c**) in the thymus following chemotherapy due to thymic rebound hyperplasia. [Thymic tissue is often reactivated post chemotherapy and is normally seen in children and young adults]

scan the patient in arms down position. Truncation artefacts are rare but difficult problems with hybrid scanner. These occur in cases where field of view of PET is larger in comparison to CT part [5].

False positives and false negatives can be countered in ^{18}F-FDG PET studies (Tables 8.3, 8.4 and 8.5). Tracer extravasation leads to false-positive tracer accumulation at the site of injection (Fig. 8.21 and 8.22). Knowledge of site of injection is

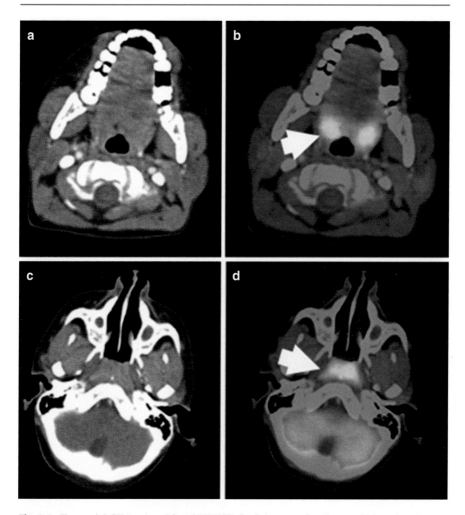

Fig. 8.8 Transaxial CT (**a, c**) and fused PET/CT (**b, d**) images of an 8-year old boy show intense symmetric uptake in normal tonsils (*arrow* in **b**) and normal adenoids (*arrow* in **d**). [Intense tracer uptake can be seen in the Waldeyer ring, especially in children, due to high physiologic activity of these lymphatic tissues and peaks at 6–8 years of age]

essential in correct interpretation of PET studies. Most of the false positives are due to infectious and inflammatory conditions [5–9]. In addition, many benign tumours may show false-positive ^{18}F-FDG uptake. Similarly some benign tumours show photopenia on PET images (Fig. 8.22 and 8.23). Small lesions beyond the resolution of PET scanners usually do not show ^{18}F-FDG uptake. Further, many cancers, such as lung carcinoid, are generally negative of ^{18}F-FDG PET studies. These false interpretations can be reduced by including CT findings in the PET/CT reports.

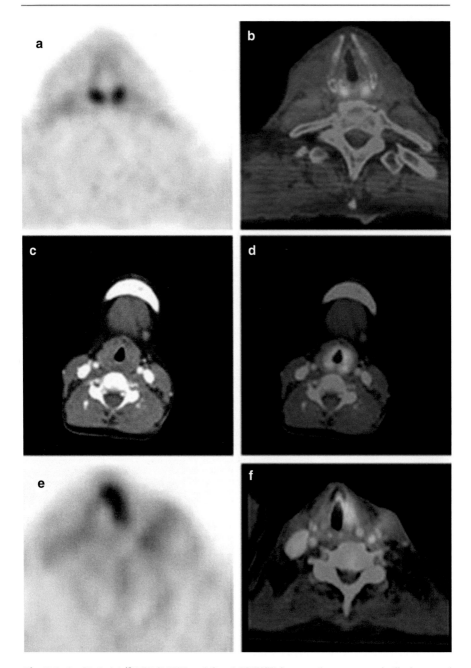

Fig. 8.9 (a, b) Axial ^{18}F-FDG PET and fused PET/CT images show symmetrically increased tracer uptake in the arytenoid muscles. (c, d) Axial CT and fused ^{18}F-FDG PET/CT images show symmetrically increased tracer uptake in the laryngeal muscles. [This should be minimised in patients with head and neck cancer by maintaining silence after tracer injection]. (e, f) Axial ^{18}F-FDG PET and fused PET/CT images show asymmetrical increased tracer uptake in the left vocal cord due to recurrent laryngeal nerve palsy on the right. [When there is asymmetrical uptake in the vocal cords, it is the normal vocal cord that demonstrates increased uptake, and the side with no increased uptake is the side with the nerve palsy]

Table 8.3 ¹⁸F-FDG scans: false-positive and false-negative tracer uptake in head/neck region [5–9, 12, 13, 16]

False positive	False negative
Physiological uptake	Small size
Brown adipose tissue (Fig. 8.10)	Recent high-dose steroid therapy
Inflammatory processes	Hyperglycaemia and hyperinsulinaemia
Post-surgical	Low-grade and well-differentiated tumours
Post-radiotherapy	Misalignment between PET and CT data
Granulomatous disease	(attenuation correction artefacts) (Fig. 8.12)
Post-chemotherapy	
Thyroiditis (Fig. 8.11)	
Benign neoplasms	
Pleomorphic adenomas	
Thyroid adenomas (Fig. 8.11)	
Salivary gland tumours	
Graves' disease (Fig. 8.11)	
Artefacts	
Misalignment between PET and CT data	
(attenuation correction artefacts)	

Table 8.4 ¹⁸F-FDG scans: false-positive and false-negative tracer uptake in the thorax [5–9, 12, 13, 16]

False positive	False negative
Physiological uptake	Small size
Brown adipose tissue (Fig. 8.10)	Recent high-dose steroid therapy
Thymus (children and young adults)	Hyperglycaemia and hyperinsulinaemia
Lactating breast and areolae (Fig. 8.2)	Low-grade and well-differentiated tumours
Skeletal and smooth muscles (Fig. 8.4)	Bronchoalveolar carcinomas
Oesophagus	Lobular carcinomas of the breast
Inflammatory processes	
Post-surgical (Fig. 8.10)	
Post-radiotherapy (Fig. 8.13)	
Post-chemotherapy (Fig. 8.13)	
Infection/inflammation (Fig. 8.14)	
Granulomatous disease (Fig. 8.13)	
Drainage tubes	
Oesophagitis (Fig. 8.14)	
Vasculitis (Fig. 8.14)	
Post-chemotherapy	
Thymic rebound hyperplasia (Fig. 8.7)	
Artefacts	
Misalignment between PET and CT data	
(attenuation correction artefacts)	

Table 8.5 ^{18}F-FDG scan: false-positive and false-negative tracer uptake in the abdomen and pelvis [5–9, 12, 13, 16]

False positive	False negative
Physiological uptake	Small size
Brown adipose tissue (Fig. 8.10)	Recent high-dose steroid therapy
Skeletal and smooth muscles (Fig. 8.4)	Hyperglycaemia and
Stomach (Fig. 8.2)	hyperinsulinaemia
Bowel (diffuse) (Fig. 8.15)	Low-grade tumours
Kidney and urinary bladder (Fig. 8.17)	Well-differentiated carcinomas
Ureters and urethra (Figs. 8.17, 8.18 and 8.19)	Hepatocellular carcinoma
Uterus during menses or corpus luteum cyst (Fig. 8.6)	Neuroendocrine tumours
Ileostomy loop (Fig. 8.17)	Mucous secreting tumours
Inflammatory processes	Prostate carcinoma
Drainage tubes	
Post-surgical (Fig. 8.16)	
Post-radiotherapy	
Post-chemotherapy	
Inflammatory bowel disease	
Cholecystitis	
Pancreatitis	
Psoas abscess	
Benign neoplasms	
Adrenal adenoma	
Ovarian cystadenoma	
Uterine fibroid (Fig. 8.20)	
Artefacts	
Misalignment between PET and CT data (attenuation correction artefacts) (Fig. 8.21)	

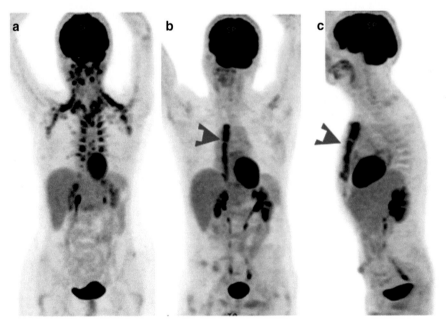

Fig. 8.10 Maximum intensity projection (MIP) ^{18}F-FDG PET images demonstrate (**a**) physiological brown fat uptake in the neck, supraclavicular fossae, mediastinum and suprarenal region and (**b**, **c**) intense tracer uptake in the sternum with recent sternotomy (*arrowheads*)

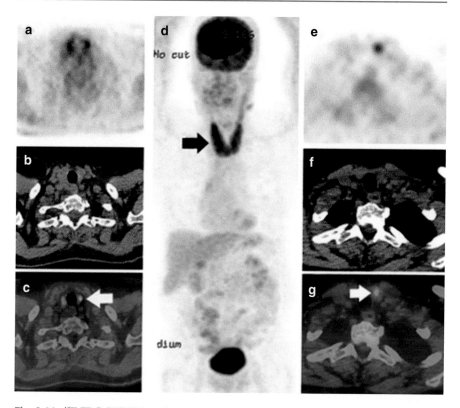

Fig. 8.11 ¹⁸F-FDG PET/CT studies: (**a–c**) transaxial PET, CT and fused images demonstrate diffuse homogenous tracer uptake in a normal size thyroid gland in a patient with known thyroiditis. (**d**) MIP image shows intense diffusely increased uptake (*arrow*) in enlarged thyroid gland in a patient with known Graves' disease. (**e–g**) Transaxial PET, CT and fused images show focal uptake (*arrow*) in the left thyroid lobe. [Diffuse uptake is seen in patients with Graves' disease, subacute thyroiditis or Hashimoto's thyroiditis, and thyroid function tests should be recommended; focal uptake in the thyroid can be malignant in approximately 1/3 of patients and should be further evaluated with ultrasound and FNA]

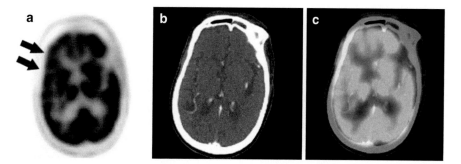

Fig. 8.12 Transaxial ¹⁸F-FDG PET (**a**), CT (**b**) and PET/CT (**c**) images of brain show apparent decreased tracer uptake in the right side of brain (*arrows*) due to head movement leading to under attenuation correction of the right side of brain

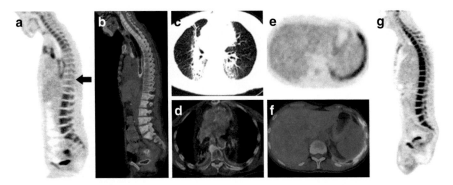

Fig. 8.13 ^{18}F-FDG PET/CT studies: (**a**, **b**) sagittal PET and fused PET/CT images show decreased tracer uptake (*arrow* in **a**) in the thoracic vertebrae due to prior radiation therapy to this site; (**c**, **d**) transaxial CT and fused PET/CT images demonstrate increased uptake in paramediastinal lung fibrosis after radiotherapy; (**e**, **f**) transaxial PET and fused PET/CT images demonstrate increased uptake in the left pleura with history of previous talc pleurodesis due to chronic granulomatous reaction [evaluation of mesothelioma is difficult following talc pleurodesis as the resulting increased pleural uptake can persist for several years]; (**g**) MIP image shows reactive diffuse tracer uptake in the bone marrow following chemotherapy in a lymphoma patient

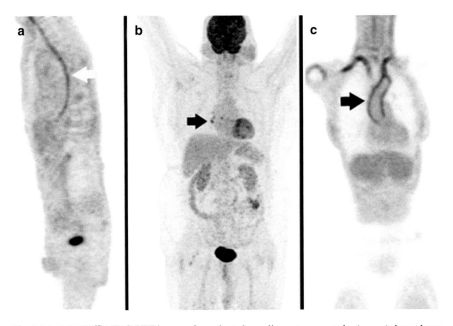

Fig. 8.14 (**a**) MIP^{18}F-FDG PET image of a patient shows linear tracer uptake (*arrow*) throughout the length of the oesophagus with no gross morphological changes suggestive of inflammatory activity. (**b**) MIP^{18}F-FDG PET image of a follow-up patient of gallbladder carcinoma shows FDG uptake in the mediastinal lymph nodes (*arrow*) with no other site of significant hypermetabolism likely due to inflammation/infection. (**c**) Coronal PET image of a patient with large vessel vasculitis shows diffusely increased FDG uptake in the wall of the aorta and its main branches (*arrow*). [If a patient is on steroids, this can result in a false-negative PET study in the evaluation of vasculitis, and ideally steroid therapy needs to be stopped for at least 3 weeks before the PET scan]

Fig. 8.15 There is diffuse uptake throughout much of the bowel, likely secondary to the patient's metformin use. [In general, patient's metformin use makes image interpretation of bowel pathology difficult]

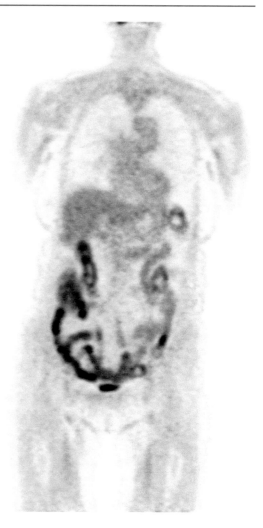

Fig. 8.16 Maximum
intensity projection (MIP)
^{18}F-FDG PET image
demonstrates intense tracer
uptake (*white arrow*) in the
anterior abdominal wall at
the site of surgical incision
in a patient with recent
open cholecystectomy.
[Increased uptake after
surgery persists for several
weeks and ideally the PET
scan should be delayed for
at least 6 weeks following
surgery]. There is also
increased uptake in the
large intestine (*black
arrow*)

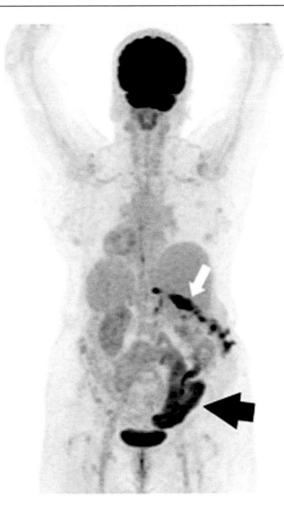

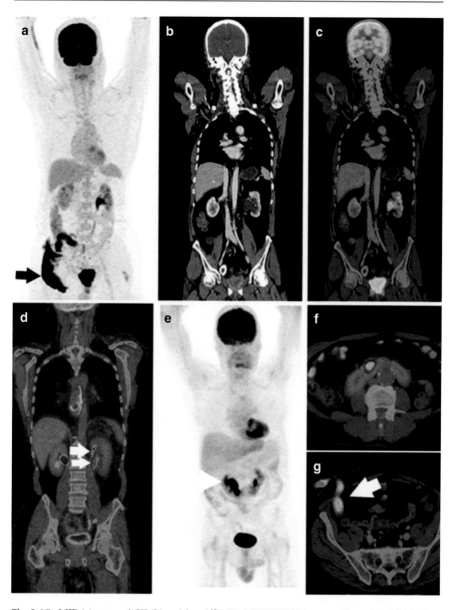

Fig. 8.17 MIP (**a**), coronal CT (**b**) and fused 18F-FDG PET/CT (**c**) images of a patient with hydronephrosis of the left kidney show tracer retention in the dilated pelvicalyceal system of the left kidney. (**a**, **g**) Intense physiological tracer uptake is also noted in the ileostomy loop (*arrow*). Coronal fused 18F-FDG PET/CT image (**d**) of a patient with duplex left kidney shows tracer uptake in two ureters (*arrows*), which may be mistaken as a lymph node in transaxial images. MIP (**e**) and transaxial fused 18F-FDG PET/CT (**f**) images of a patient with horseshoe kidney show tracer activity within the fused kidneys in the midline of the abdomen

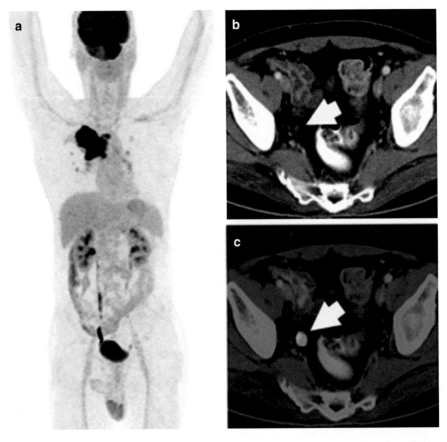

Fig. 8.18 Tracer uptake in the dilated ureter may mimic a lymph node (*arrows* in **b**, **c**). [Correlation of tracer activity on the MIP image (**a**) and following the ureter on transaxial images are helpful]

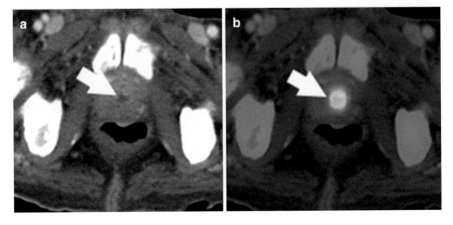

Fig. 8.19 Physiological intense focal urinary tracer activity in the prostatic urethra (*arrows* in **a**, **b**) in a patient with adenocarcinoma of prostate following transurethral resection of the prostate. [Most prostate cancers are not FDG avid; however, approximately 10–15 % of incidental focal prostate uptake is related to malignancy, and if seen, biochemical evaluation with serum PSA is advised]

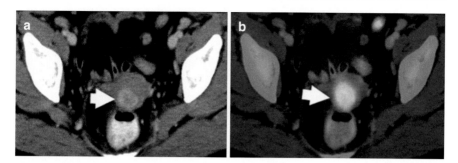

Fig. 8.20 Intense tracer uptake is seen in an enhancing soft tissue lesion in the uterine wall (*arrows* in **a**, **b**) suggestive of fibroid. [Any increased uptake in the uterus in a postmenopausal woman should be investigated and an ultrasound is advised in the first instance]

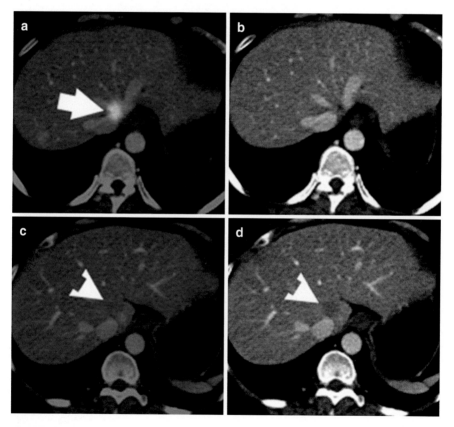

Fig. 8.21 Misregistration: transaxial fused ¹⁸F-FDG PET/CT and CT images show a hypodense hepatic lesion (*arrowhead* in **c**, **d**) that has been misplaced to slightly higher level during PET image acquisition (*arrow* in **a**) due to differences in breathing patterns between CT and PET image acquisitions. Note there is no lesion on CT image (**b**) corresponding to apparent site of tracer uptake on fused image (*arrow* in **a**). [In general, motion artefacts, reconstruction artefacts and noise are usually self-evident in most cases]

Fig. 8.22 MIP ^{18}F-FDG
PET image shows tracer
extravasation at the site of
injection (*arrows*). [A local
view of the extravasation
site is often undertaken to
establish what proportion
of the administered activity
remains at the
extravasation site. The
SUV measurements will
also be affected]

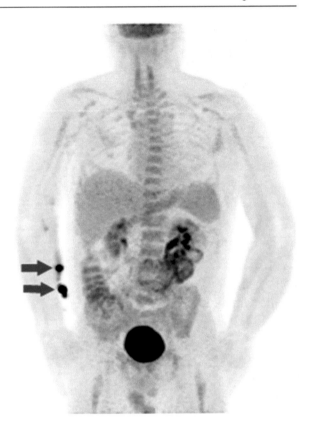

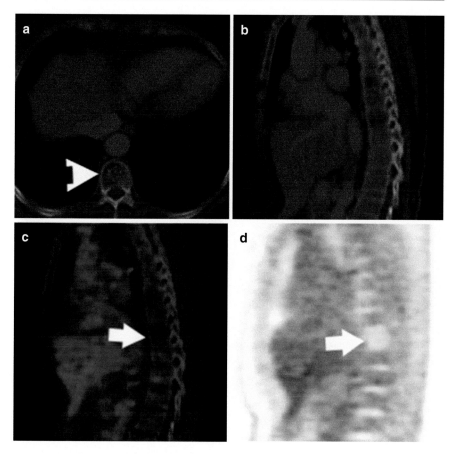

Fig. 8.23 Sagittal CT, fused and PET (**b, c, d**) images show Focal photopenia (*arrows* in **c, d**) in a vertebral haemangioma showing "polka-dot appearance" on corresponding transaxial CT image (*arrowhead* in **a**). [Vertebral haemangiomata can be "hot" or "cold" on FDG PET imaging]

Conclusions

It is vital to recognise the normal variants and artefacts for accurate interpretation of ^{18}F-FDG PET/CT studies. Furthermore, recognising false positive and false negatives is equally important for correct interpretation of PET/CT findings.

Key Points

- ^{18}F-FDG is transported into cells through glucose transporters and phosphorylated by enzyme hexokinase to ^{18}F-FDG-6-phosphate.
- ^{18}F-FDG is accumulated in malignant tissues more avidly than within the normal tissues.

- ^{18}F-FDG PET/CT scans often show variable degrees of physiological tracer uptake in various organs.
- Recognition of physiological tracer distribution is essential in avoiding wrong image interpretation.
- It is vital to recognise normal variants and artefacts to avoid misinterpretation
- Misregistration is noted due to differences in breathing patterns and patient movement between CT and PET image acquisitions. It is vital to recognise misregistration to avoid misinterpretation.
- False positives and false negatives can be countered in 18F-FDG PET studies.
- ^{18}F-FDG uptake is known to occur in inflammation, infection and healing tissues.
- ^{18}F-FDG PET study immediately after chemotherapy and radiotherapy may introduce false-positive findings.
- Recognising false positive and false negatives is important for accurate reporting.

Acknowledgements Thanks to Dr. Nerriman, Dr. Riyamma and Dr. Halsey for contributing images for the chapter on "PET/CT Imaging: Normal variants, Pitfalls and Artefacts".

References

1. Agrawal K, Mittal BR, Bansal D, et al. Role of F-18 FDG PET/CT in assessing bone marrow involvement in pediatric Hodgkin's lymphoma. Ann Nucl Med. 2013;27(2):146–51.
2. Mittal BR, Agrawal K. FDG-PET in tuberculosis. Curr Mol Imaging. 2014;3(3):211–5.
3. Cook GJR, Fogelman I, Maisey MN. Normal physiological and benign pathological variants of ^{18}F-FDG PET scanning: potential for error in interpretation. Semin Nucl Med. 1996;26: 308–14.
4. Cook GJR, Maisey MN, Fogelman I. Normal variants, artefacts and interpretative pitfalls in PET imaging with ^{18}F-fluoro-2-deoxyglucose and carbon-11 methionine. Eur J Nucl Med. 1999;26:1363–78.
5. Cook GJ, Wegner EA, Fogelman I. Pitfalls and artifacts in 18FDG PET and PET/CT oncologic imaging. Semin Nucl Med. 2004;34:122–33.
6. Culverwell AD, Scarsbrook AF, Chowdhury FU. False-positive uptake on 2-[^{18}F]-fluoro-2-deoxy-D-glucose (FDG) positron-emission tomography/computed tomography (PET/CT) in oncological imaging. Clin Radiol. 2011;66:366–82.
7. Shreve PD, Anzai Y, Wahl RL. Pitfalls in oncologic diagnosis with FDG PET imaging: physiologic and benign variants. Radiographics. 1999;19:61–77.
8. Delbeke D, Coleman RE, Guiberteau MJ, et al. Procedure guideline for tumour imaging with ^{18}F-FDG PET/CT 1.0. J Nucl Med. 2006;47:885–95.
9. Boellaard R, O'Doherty MJ, Weber WA, et al. FDG PET and PET/CT: EANM procedure guidelines for tumour PET imaging: version 1.0. Eur J Nucl Med Mol Imaging. 2010;37: 181–200.
10. Segall G, Delbeke D, Stabin MG, et al. SNM practice guideline for sodium 18F-fluoride PET/CT bone scans 1.0. J Nucl Med. 2010;51:1813–20.

11. Juweid ME, Cheson BD. Positron-emission tomography and assessment of cancer therapy. N Engl J Med. 2006;354:496–507.
12. Gorospe L, Raman S, Echeveste J, et al. Whole-body PET/CT: spectrum of physiological variants, artifacts and interpretative pitfalls in cancer patients. Nucl Med Commun. 2005;26: 671–87.
13. Shammas A, Lim R, Charron M. Pediatric FDG PET/CT: physiologic uptake, normal variants, and benign conditions. Radiographics. 2009;29:1467–86.
14. Harisankar CN, Mittal BR, Agrawal KL, et al. Utility of high fat and low carbohydrate diet in suppressing myocardial FDG uptake. J Nucl Cardiol. 2011;18:926–36.
15. Agrawal K, Weaver J, Ngu R, et al. Clinical significance of patterns of incidental thyroid uptake at (18)F-FDG PET/CT. Clin Radiol. 2015;70(5):536–43.
16. Corrigan AJ, Schleyer PJ, Cook GJ. Pitfalls and artifacts in the use of PET/CT in oncology imaging. Semin Nucl Med. 2015;45(6):481–99.

FDG-PET/CT in Oesophageal and Gastric Cancer

9

Teresa A. Szyszko

Contents

9.1 Indications for PET/CT

Oesophageal and gastric malignancy are considered together in the RCR-RCP guidelines for FDG-PET/CT imaging in the UK. Indications for use of FDG-PET/CT imaging in oesophagogastric malignancy include staging/restaging of patients suitable for radical treatment, including patients who have received neoadjuvant treatment [1]. It also may be indicated in suspected recurrence, when other imaging is negative or equivocal, as biological changes in the tumour usually precede morphological changes.

T.A. Szyszko
King's College and Guy's and St Thomas' PET Centre, Division of Imaging Sciences and Biomedical Engineering, Kings College London, St Thomas' Hospital, London, UK
e-mail: teresa.szyszko-walls@kcl.ac.uk

© Springer International Publishing Switzerland 2016
T.A. Szyszko (ed.), *PET/CT in Oesophageal and Gastric Cancer*, Clinicians' Guides to Radionuclide Hybrid Imaging, DOI 10.1007/978-3-319-29240-3_9

9.2   Staging of Oesophageal Cancer

9.2.1   T-Stage Evaluation

FDG-PET has a limited role in T staging. Although it is sensitive in detecting both squamous cell lesions in the proximal oesophagus and adenocarcinomas in the distal ocsophagus and gastro-oesophageal junction [2] and has the added advantage of accurate localisation of lesions [3], its value is limited by its low spatial resolution. It may fail to detect small primary oesophageal lesions (5–8 mm) and hence sensitivity is reduced in detecting early-stage (stage 1 and 2) disease. In one study (Kato et al.) [4], this was as low as 43 % in stage 1 tumours. It does, however, have better sensitivity in identifying advanced disease; especially stage 4 [3]. Hence the overall sensitivity was 80 % [4].

Sensitivity of FDG-PET is also reduced in non-FDG-avid oesophageal tumours such as well- differentiated tumours (with low GLUT 1 expression) and mucus-secreting tumours [5]. Gastro-oesophageal reflux or physiological smooth muscle oesophageal uptake can cause false-positive results [6].

Interestingly, the SUVmax measurement in the primary tumour has prognostic value in that multivariate analysis has shown a significant difference in overall survival and response ($p < 0.05$) in patients undergoing chemoradiotherapy where the SUVmax in the primary tumour is <10 and in those where it is ≥ 10 [7]. Other prognostic factors include total lesion glycolysis (TLG), metastatic length of disease (MLoD) and total lymph node count (PET/CT LNMC) [8].

9.2.2   N-Stage Evaluation

FDG-PET/CT is a useful tool in evaluating nodal disease, although uptake in locoregional nodes is often hampered by uptake in the primary tumour itself. Locoregional nodes include any paraoesophageal nodes extending from cervical nodes to coeliac nodes. These include supraclavicular and left gastric nodes (Appendix 1). The stage depends on the number of involved nodes ($N0 = 0$; $N1 = 1–2$; $N2 = 3–6$; $N3 \geq 7$). The main advantage of PET is in identifying disease in normal-sized lymph nodes and differentiating between inflammatory and metastatic enlarged lymph nodes [4], thus limiting the need for invasive procedures such as mediastinoscopy [3]. Many studies have shown that the diagnostic sensitivity specificity and accuracy for PET in detection of individual lymph node metastases are significantly better than CT [4, 9] (Fig. 9.1).

A meta-analysis of FDG-PET in staging oesophageal cancer showed that it had a sensitivity of 57 % but high specificity of 85 % [10]. A more recent meta-analysis of nodal staging with PET/CT rather than PET revealed similar findings with PET/CT resulting in a sensitivity of 55–62 % but specificity of 76–96 % [11]. EUS was been shown to have slightly higher sensitivity that PET/CT in identifying locoregional disease [12] and EUS results have shown accuracy in the range of 75 % for initial staging of regional lymph nodes [13].

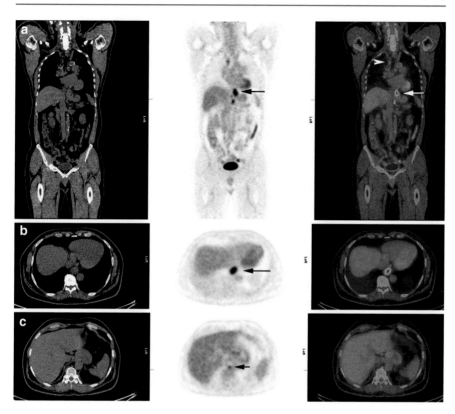

Fig. 9.1 (**a**) Coronal image of low-dose CT, PET and fused PET/CT in a 69-year-old patient with newly diagnosed adenocarcinoma extending from the distal oesophagus into the cardia of the stomach which demonstrates high-grade uptake in the primary lesion (*black arrow*) but also uptake in mediastinal and upper abdominal lymph nodes in keeping with widespread nodal disease (*white arrows*). (**b**) Axial image in the same patient showing thickening of the oesophageal wall (*black arrow*) with increased FDG uptake (SUVmax = 10.7) at the site of the primary lesion. (**c**) Axial image in the same patient demonstrating uptake in a small retrocrural lymph node (*black arrow*) which is also likely to be involved in the disease process. This would not be identified on the CT alone

The lower sensitivity of FDG-PET/CT may be due to the limited ability of PET in detecting nodal disease in the direct vicinity of the primary lesion where the uptake in the tumour may obscure peritumoural nodes, resulting in a false negative [14, 15]. In addition, limited spatial resolution and microscopic metastatic disease within lymph nodes may also result on false-negative findings [16]. False-positive findings are unusual and may be due to granulomatous disorders.

9.2.3   M-Stage Evaluation

The undisputed value of FDG-PET/CT is in evaluating distant metastases where PET is highly sensitive, accurate and cost effective in comparison to CT and EUS [3]

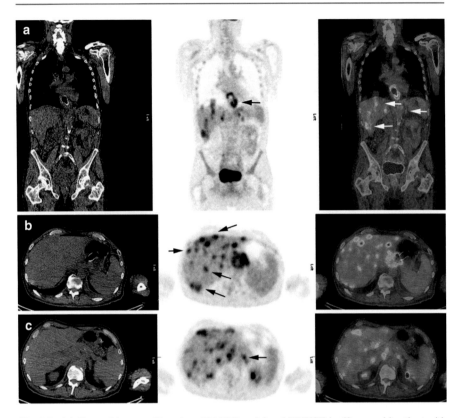

Fig. 9.2 (**a**) Coronal image of low-dose CT, PET and fused PET/CT in 62-year-old patient with newly diagnosed squamous cell carcinoma of the lower oesophagus demonstrates high-grade uptake in the primary lesion (*black arrow*) but also multiple distant metastases (*white arrows*). (**b**) Axial image in the same patient showing uptake is seen in multiple liver metastases (*black arrows*). (**c**) Axial image in the same patient demonstrating uptake in a metastasis in the medial limb of the left adrenal gland (*black arrow*)

Distant metastases are present in 20–30 % of oesophageal tumours at initial staging [17]. PET/CT allows detection of metastatic disease, which may not be identifiable with other methods (Fig. 9.2). It has been shown to improve preoperative staging and prevent inappropriate intervention, and even in patients not suitable for surgery, the detection of unsuspected metastases can guide palliative management [18].

The most common sites for metastatic disease are nonregional nodes, such as nodes at the porta hepatis and retroperitoneal nodes, and organ metastases to the lungs, liver, bones and adrenals [19, 20]. These are now all considered as M1 disease, and the subclassifications of M1a, M1b and Mx are no longer used. However, PET/CT also has a high sensitivity for detecting metastases which occur in unexpected locations and can be radiologically occult. These include metastases to the brain, skeletal muscle, subcutaneous tissue, thyroid gland and pancreas [4, 21]. Its sensitivity and accuracy are greater than EUS and CT combined in detecting supraclavicular and retroperitoneal nodal disease [22]. This prospective study also showed that PET/CT revealed unsuspected disease in 17% patients who were refereed for nonsurgical workup. PET/CT upstaged 15% patients from M0 to M1, especially those with T3 tumours and downstaged 7% from M1 to M0. This was confirmed in another prospective study which showed that PET/CT correctly upstaged 20% and downstaged 5% patients sparing unnecessary surgery in those with disseminated disease [23].

FDG-PET/CT has high sensitivity and specificity in detecting oesophageal metastases. A large meta-analysis of FDG-PET only data concluded that for the evaluation of distant metastases, FDG-PET had a higher sensitivity than CT alone [10]. This diminishes with smaller lesions; however even very small lesions which demonstrate high metabolically are seen. The specificity of PEt alone is also high (90–98%) [3]. False positives can be caused by inflammation and physiological bowel uptake. A comparison of PET with PET/CT showed that PET/CT had an incremental value over PEt alone, especially in cervical disease [24], and provides superior accuracy due to precise localisation of metabolic activity [3].

PET/CT can also detect unsuspected synchronous tumours, which occur in 5.5% of patients with oesophageal malignancy [25]. These most commonly occur in the stomach, head and neck and colon [18] but have also been found in the kidney, thyroid and lung [25].

9.3   Treatment Response in Oesophageal Cancer

There have been mixed results in the use of PET for assessment of treatment response. Post-radiotherapy oesophagitis can also demonstrate significant uptake and it is important to wait 8–12 weeks post radiotherapy to avoid false positives [18]. Postoperative inflammation can also result in false positives and hence it is important to wait 4–6 weeks post surgery to avoid this.

FDG decrease after therapy in responders has been shown to correlate closely to histopathological outcome and a pathologic response within tumour has been reported to correspond to decreases in SUV max of 35–60% between initial staging PET and re-evaluation imaging [26–30]. It is can be a means of evaluating treatment response [2] and can identify responders to neoadjuvant therapy [31]. Persistent FDG uptake (with an SUV ≥ 4) on a single post-treatment scan has been shown to correlate with residual tumour and poor survival [32]. However, recent studies have found that post-treatment PET/CT can be prone to false positives due to post treatment oesophagitis and ulceration [33]. Radiation oesophagitis is seen after the first weeks of treatment [34] and is more common with higher radiation doses.

The timing of the post-treatment PET/CT is also important. In most studies, PET/CT has been performed at the end of treatment. However, Weber et al. found that PET/CT performed after two cycles of chemotherapy allowed prediction of long-term outcome with a sensitivity and specificity of 93 and 95%, respectively [35], suggesting there may be a more useful role for PET/CT in early treatment monitoring, especially of this can be performed within the first 2 weeks of treatment, before oesophagitis has had time to develop.

Respiratory motion artefact is greatest at the level of the diaphragm and hence distal oesophageal and gastro-oesophageal tumours are especially prone to this artefact which can alter SUVmax measurements by up to 30–50 % [36]. This is a further source of potential error when looking at treatment response with PET/CT.

Whilst PET/CT is recommended to improve the accuracy of M staging for patients who are potential candidates for curative therapy, there is no recommendation for or against use of PET/CT for the assessment of treatment response, due to insufficient evidence [37]. However, identification of PET-positive lymph nodes after completion of chemotherapy is a predictor of poor prognosis in patients scheduled for surgery and FDG-PET lymph node status after neoadjuvant chemotherapy is more important than that before chemotherapy [38].

A recent study looking at restaging oesophageal cancer after neoadjuvant therapy with FDG PET-CT found that it is more sensitive than CT for detecting interval progression and identifies metastases in 6 % of patients. Despite this, at surgery 10 % of patients had unsuspected incurable disease. FDG-avid nodal stage before chemotherapy plus tumour FDG-avid length predicted subsequent progression [39].

Key Points
Oesophageal Cancer

- Indications for use of FDG-PET/CT imaging in oesophagogastric malignancy include staging/restaging of patients suitable for radical treatment, including patients who have received neoadjuvant treatment.
- FDG-PET/CT may be indicated in suspected recurrence, when other imaging is negative or equivocal.
- FDG-PET has a limited role in T staging.
- FDG-PET may fail to detect small primary oesophageal lesions (5–8 mm) and hence sensitivity is reduced in detecting early-stage disease.
- FDG-PET sensitivity is reduced in non-FDG-avid oesophageal tumours (well-differentiated and mucus-secreting tumours).
- Gastro-oesophageal reflux or physiological smooth muscle oesophageal uptake can cause false-positive results on FDG-PET.
- FDG-PET/CT is a useful tool in evaluating nodal disease (although uptake in locoregional nodes is often hampered by uptake in the primary tumour itself).
- The main advantage of PET is in identifying disease in normal-sized lymph nodes and differentiating between inflammatory and metastatic enlarged lymph nodes.
- FDG-PET/CT useful in evaluating distant metastases where PET is highly sensitive, accurate and cost effective in comparison to CT and EUS.
- There have been mixed results in the use of PET for assessment of treatment response

9.4 Gastric Cancer

Only a few published studies have evaluated gastric cancer with FDG-PET. Limitations for the use of PET/CT include physiological uptake in gastric mucosa which may be significant causing difficulty in identifying tumours. Low FDG uptake also occurs in signet ring and mucinous tumours. FDG uptake in small tumours is underestimated due to partial value averaging. Intestinal-type tumours have higher uptake than diffuse type [38].

As with oesophageal malignancy, the role of PET/CT is limited in gastric malignancy T staging and this is best evaluated with EUS. The low spatial resolution of FDG-PET makes it less sensitive than CT in the detection of local perigastric nodes. However, PET/CT has a high specificity for detecting lymph node metastases [40]. In advanced gastric cancer, GLUT-1 expression and Ki-67 labelling index are important factors in predicting FDG uptake in metastatic lymph nodes [41]. PET, once again, is most valuable in the detection of distant metastases, such as those to the liver, lungs, adrenal glands, ovaries, bone and distant nodal metastases. A few studies have reported that PET may be useful in the detection of peritoneal metastases [42–44]. These may appear as diffuse uptake spreading uniformly throughout the abdomen and pelvis, obscuring visceral outline, or as random discrete foci of uptake [44, 45]. For peritoneal metastases, PET/CT has a poorer sensitivity of 35 % but better specificity of 99 % than CT [46].

PET may also be helpful in the follow-up of patients undergoing chemotherapy as it allows early identification of response to treatment [47]. There are only a few studies using FDG-PET/CT to predict response to neoadjuvant or adjuvant chemotherapy. A complete metabolic response seems to be predictive of a more favourable prognosis.

9.5 Gastrointestinal Stromal Tumours (GIST)

In staging gastrointestinal stromal tumours (GIST), FDG-PET/CT is indicated prior to treatment in patients who are likely to require systemic therapy and also in response assessment to systemic therapy [1].

GISTs are mesenchymal in origin and account for less than 1 % of gastric tumours. A comparison of FDG-PET and CT in staging and evaluation of treatment response to imatinib mesylate therapy in recurrent or metastatic GIST showed that PET and CT were comparable in staging; however, FDG-PET was superior to CT in predicting early response to treatment [48]. Further studies have also shown convincing evidence that serial PET study is more sensitive and reliable for determining treatment response to imatinib mesylate in patients of GIST, when compared with only conventional CT monitoring, and that PET appears to be of potential value in initial disease evaluation including prediction of malignant potential in recently diagnosed GIST and in selection of optimal dose of imatinib for therapy [49].

9.6   Radiotherapy Planning

Use of PET/CT in radiotherapy planning in oesophageal cancer seems to positively contribute to target volume delineation. When compared to CT-based radiotherapy planning, changes in primary tumour length were observed in 75–86 % patients and changes in gross tumour volume (GTV) were observed in 59–100 % [50–52]. When using 4D FDG-PET/CT to delineate GTV, a SUV threshold setting of 20 % or SUV 2.5 achieves the optimal correlation of tumour length, volume ratio and conformality index [53]. Rapid oesophageal tumour progression has been demonstrated in the interval between diagnostic FDG-PET and FDG-PET for radiotherapy planning and hence this should be kept to a minimum [54].

Key Points to Remember
Gastric Cancer
- Physiological FDG-PET uptake in gastric mucosa may cause difficulty in identifying grade tumours.
- Intestinal-type tumours have higher 18F-FDG uptake than diffuse.
- PET/CT is limited in gastric malignancy T staging and this is best evaluated with EUS (less sensitive than CT in the detection of local perigastric nodes).
- PET/CT has a high specificity for detecting lymph node metastases.
- In peritoneal metastases, PET/CT has a poorer sensitivity of 35 % but better specificity of 99 % than CT.
- PET may also be helpful in the follow-up of patients undergoing chemotherapy as it allows early identification of response to treatment.
- FDG-PET/CT is indicated prior to treatment in patients with GIST who are likely to require systemic therapy and also in response assessment to systemic therapy.
- PET/CT in radiotherapy planning in oesophageal cancer seems to positively contribute to target volume delineation.

PET/CT in oesophagogastric malignancy	T stage	N stage	M stage
Advantage	Better sensitivity in staging advanced rather than early-stage disease but less sensitive than EUS Useful in staging and treatment response in GIST	Identifying disease in normal-sized lymph nodes Differentiating between metastatic and inflammatory nodes Better than CT but less sensitive than EUS	Main advantage of PET/CT Highly sensitive, specific, accurate and cost effective Detects radiologically occult disease

PET/CT in oesophagogastric malignancy	T stage	N stage	M stage
Limitations	Small lesions Well-differentiated tumours Mucus-secreting tumours	Uptake in primary tumour may obscure peritumoural nodes Microscopic nodal metastases	Sensitivity diminishes with smaller lesions but even small metabolically active lesions are detected
Pitfalls	Low sensitivity in early-stage disease Physiological GI uptake Persistent uptake in post-radiotherapy oesophagitis resulting in false positive	False positive in granulomatous disease	False positive in inflammation

References

1. Barrington S, Scarsbrook A, The Royal College of Physicians and the Royal College of Radiologists. Evidence-based indications for the use of PETCT in the UK. London: RCP, RCR; 2013.
2. Kostakoglu L, Agress Jr H, Stanley J. Goldsmith clinical role of FDG PET in evaluation of cancer patients. Radiographics. 2003;23(2):315–40.
3. Marzola MC, De Manzoni G, Grassetto G, Cordiano C, Al-Nahhas A, Alavi A, Rubello D. Extended staging of oesophageal cancer using FDG-PET – a critical appraisal. Eur J Radiol. 2012;81(1):21–30.
4. Kato H, Miyazaki T, Nakajima M, Takita J, Kimura H, Faried A, et al. The incremental effect of positron emission tomography on diagnostic accuracy in the initial staging of esophageal carcinoma. Cancer. 2005;103(1):148–56.
5. Flamen P. Positron emission tomography in gastric and esophageal cancer. Curr Opin Oncol. 2004;16(4):359–63.
6. Bruzzi JF, Truong MT, Marom EM, Mawlawi O, Podoloff DA, Macapinlac HA, Munden RF. Incidental findings on integrated PET/CT that do not accumulate 18F-FDG. AJR Am J Roentgenol. 2006;187(4):1116–23.
7. Atsumi K, Nakamura K, Abe K, Hirakawa M, Shioyama Y, Sasaki T, et al. Prediction of outcome with FDG-PET in definitive chemoradiotherapy for esophageal cancer. J Radiat Res. 2013;54(5):890–8.
8. Foley KG, Fielding P, Lewis WG, Karran A, Chan D, Blake P, Roberts SA. Prognostic significance of novel ^{18}F-FDG PET/CT defined tumour variables in patients with oesophageal cancer. Eur J Radiol. 2014;83(7):1069–73.
9. Rankin SC, Taylor H, Cook GJ, Mason R. Computed tomography and positron emission tomography in the pre-operative staging of oesophageal carcinoma. Clin Radiol. 1998;53(9):659–65.
10. Van Vliet E, Heijenbrok-Kal MH, Hunink MG, Kuipers EJ, Siersema PD. Staging investigations for oesophageal cancer: a meta-analysis. Br J Cancer. 2008;98:547–57.
11. Shi W, Wang W, Wang J, Cheng H, Huo X. Meta-analysis of 18 FDG PET-CT for nodal staging in patients with esophageal cancer. Surg Oncol. 2013;22(2):112–6.
12. Walker AJ, Spier BJ, Perlman SB, Stangl JR, Frick TJ, Gopal DV, et al. Integrated PET/CT fusion imaging and endoscopic ultrasound in the pre-operative staging and evaluation of esophageal cancer. Mol Imaging Biol. 2011;13(1):166–71.

13. Lightdale CJ, Kulkarni KG. Role of endoscopic ultrasonography in the staging and follow-up of esophageal cancer. J Clin Oncol. 2005;23(20):4483–9.
14. Yoon HH, Lowe VJ, Cassivi SD, Romero Y. The role of FDG-PET and staging laparoscopy in the management of patients with cancer of the esophagus or gastroesophageal junction. Gastroenterol Clin North Am. 2009;38(1):105–20.
15. Dehdashti F, Siegel BA. Neoplasms of the esophagus and stomach. Semin Nucl Med. 2004;34(3):198–208.
16. Lerut T, Flamen P, Fctors N, Van Cutsem E, Peeters M, Hiele M, et al. Histopathologic validation of lymph node staging with FDG-PET scan in cancer of the esophagus and gastroesophageal junction: a prospective study based on primary surgery with extensive lymphadenectomy. Ann Surg. 2000;232(6):743–52.
17. Flanagan FL, Dehdashti F, Siegel BA, Trask DD, Sundaresan SR, Patterson GA, Cooper JD. Staging of esophageal cancer with 18F-fluorodeoxyglucose positron emission tomography. AJR Am J Roentgenol. 1997;168(2):417–24.
18. Bruzzi JF, Munden RF, Truong MT, Marom EM, Sabloff BS, Gladish GW, Iyer RB, Pan TS, Macapinlac HA, Erasmus JJ. PET/CT of esophageal cancer: its role in clinical management. Radiographics. 2007;27(6):1635–52.
19. Roth JA, Putnam Jr JB, Rich T, Forastiere AA. Cancer of the esophagus. In: DeVita Jr VT, Hellman S, Rosenberg SA, editors. Cancer: principles and practice of oncology. 5th ed. New York: Lippincott-Raven; 1997. p. 980–1021.
20. Quint LE, Hepburn LM, Francis IR, Whyte RI, Orringer MB. Incidence and distribution of distant metastases from newly diagnosed esophageal carcinoma. Cancer. 1995;76:1120–5.
21. Bruzzi JF, Truong MT, Macapinlac H, Munden RF, Erasmus JJ. Integrated CT-PET imaging of esophageal cancer: unexpected and unusual distribution of distant organ metastases. Curr Probl Diagn Radiol. 2007;36:21–9.
22. Flamen P, Lerut A, Van Cutsem E, De Wever W, Peeters M, Stroobants S. Utility of positron emission tomography for the staging of patients with potentially operable esophageal carcinoma. J Clin Oncol. 2000;18:3202–10.
23. Heeren P, Jager PL, Bongaerts F, van Dullemen H, Sluiter W, Plukker JT. Detection of distant metastases in esophageal cancer with 18F FDG PET. J Nucl Med. 2004;45:980–7.
24. Bar-Shalom R, Guralnik L, Tsalic M, Leiderman M, Frenkel A, Gaitini D, et al. The additional value of PET/CT over PET in FDG imaging of oesophageal cancer. Eur J Nucl Med Mol Imaging. 2005;32(8):918–24.
25. Van Westreenen HL, Westerterp M, Jager PL, van Dullemen HM, Sloof GW, Comans EF, et al. Synchronous primary neoplasms detected on 18F-FDG PET in staging of patients with esophageal cancer. J Nucl Med. 2005;46(8):1321–5.
26. Downey RJ, Akhurst T, Ilson D, et al. Whole body 18FDG-PET and the response of esophageal cancer to induction therapy: results of a prospective trial. J Clin Oncol. 2003;21:428–32.
27. Flamen P, Van Cutsem E, Lerut A, et al. Positron emission tomography for assessment of the response to induction radiochemotherapy in locally advanced oesophageal cancer. Ann Oncol. 2002;13:361–8.
28. Wieder HA, Brucher BL, Zimmermann F, et al. Time course of tumor metabolic activity during chemoradiotherapy of esophageal squamous cell carcinoma and response to treatment. J Clin Oncol. 2004;22:900–8.
29. Kroep JR, Van Groeningen CJ, Cuesta MA, et al. Positron emission tomography using 2-deoxy-2-[18F]-fluoro-D-glucose for response monitoring in locally advanced gastroesophageal cancer: a comparison of different analytical methods. Mol Imaging Biol. 2003;5:337–46.
30. Brucher BL, Weber W, Bauer M, et al. Neoadjuvant therapy of esophageal squamous cell carcinoma: response evaluation by positron emission tomography. Ann Surg. 2001;233:300–9.
31. Kelly S, Harris KM, Berry E, et al. A systematic review of the staging performance of endoscopic ultrasound in gastro-oesophageal carcinoma. Gut. 2001;49:534–9.

32. Kato H, Kuwano H, Nakajima M, et al. Usefulness of positron emission tomography for assessing the response of neoadjuvant chemoradiotherapy in patients with esophageal cancer. Am J Surg. 2002;184:279–83.
33. Erasmus JJ, Munden RF, Truong MT, et al. Pre-operative chemoradiation-induced ulceration in patients with esophageal cancer: a confounding factor in tumor response assessment in integrated CT-PET imaging. J Thorac Oncol. 2006;1:478–86.
34. Hautzel H, Müller-Gärtner HW. Early changes in fluorine-18-FDG uptake during radiotherapy. J Nucl Med. 1997;38(9):1384–6.
35. Weber WA, Ott K, Becker K, Dittler HJ, Helmberger H, Avril NE, et al. Prediction of response to preoperative chemotherapy in adenocarcinomas of the esophagogastric junction by metabolic imaging. J Clin Oncol. 2001;19(12):3058–65.
36. Pan T, Mawlawi O, Nehmeh SA, et al. Attenuation correction of PET images with respiration-averaged CT images in PET/CT. J Nucl Med. 2005;46:1481–7.
37. Wong R, Walker-Dilks C, Raifu A. Evidence-based guideline recommendations on the use of positron emission tomography imaging in oesophageal cancer. Clin Oncol (R Coll Radiol). 2012;24(2):86–104.
38. Miyata H, Yamasaki M, Takahashi T, Murakami K, Kurokawa Y, Nakajima K, et al. Relevance of [18F]fluorodeoxyglucose positron emission tomography-positive lymph nodes after neoadjuvant chemotherapy for squamous cell oesophageal cancer. Br J Surg. 2013;100(11):1490–7.
39. Findlay JM, Gillies RS, Franklin JM, Teoh EJ, Jones GE, di Carlo S, et al Restaging oesophageal cancer after neoadjuvant therapy with (18) F-FDG PET-CT: identifying interval metastases and predicting incurable disease at surgery. Eur Radiol. 2016 Feb 16. [Epub ahead of print]
40. Yun M. Imaging of gastric cancer metabolism using 18 F-FDG PET/CT. J Gastric Cancer. 2014;14(1):1–6.
41. Kim YH, Choi JY, Do IG, Kim S, Kim BT. Factors affecting 18F-FDG uptake by metastatic lymph nodes in gastric cancer. J Comput Assist Tomogr. 2013;37(5):815–9.
42. Kluge R, Schmidt F, Caca K, et al. Positron emission tomography with [(18)F]fluoro-2-deoxydglucose for diagnosis and staging of bile duct cancer. Hepatology. 2001;33:1029–35.
43. Tanaka T, Kawai Y, Kanai M, Taki Y, Nakamoto Y, Takabayashi A. Usefulness of FDG-positron emission tomography in diagnosing peritoneal recurrence of colorectal cancer. Am J Surg. 2002;184:433–6.
44. Turlakow A, Yeung HW, Salmon AS, Macapinlac HA, Larson SM. Peritoneal carcinomatosis: roleof (18)F-FDG PET. J Nucl Med. 2003;44:1407–12.
45. Lin EC, Lear J, Quaife RA. Metastatic peritoneal seeding patterns demonstrated by FDG positronemission tomographic imaging. Clin Nucl Med. 2001;26:249–50.
46. Lim JS, Kim MJ, Yun MJ, Oh YT, Kim JH, Hwang HS, et al. Comparison of CT and 18F-FDG pet for detecting peritoneal metastasis on the preoperative evaluation for gastric carcinoma. Korean J Radiol. 2006;7:249–56.
47. Lim JS, Yun MJ, Kim MJ, Hyung WJ, Park MS, Choi JY, et al. CT and PET in stomach cancer: preoperative staging and monitoring of response to therapy. Radiographics. 2006;26(1):143–56.
48. Gayed I, Vu T, Iyer R, Johnson M, Macapinlac H, Swanston N, Podoloff D. The role of 18F-FDG PET in staging and early prediction of response to therapy of recurrent gastrointestinal stromal tumors. J Nucl Med. 2004;45(1):17–21.
49. Basu S, Mohandas KM, Peshwe H, Asopa R, Vyawahare M. FDG-PET and PET/CT in the clinical management of gastrointestinal stromal tumor. Nucl Med Commun. 2008;29(12):1026–39.
50. Moureau-Zabotto L, Touboul E, Lerouge D, Deniaud-Alexandre E, Grahek D, Foulquier JN, et al. Impact of CT and 18F-deoxyglucose positron emission tomography image fusion for conformal radiotherapy in esophageal carcinoma. Int J Radiat Oncol Biol Phys. 2005;63(2):340–5.

51. Muijs CT, Schreurs LM, Busz DM, Beukema JC, van der Borden AJ, Pruim J, et al. Consequences of additional use of PET information for target volume delineation and radiotherapy dose distribution for esophageal cancer. Radiother Oncol. 2009;93(3):447–53.
52. Schreurs LM, Busz DM, Paardekooper GM, Beukema JC, Jager PL, Van der Jagt EJ, et al. Impact of 18-fluorodeoxyglucose positron emission tomography on computed tomography defined target volumes in radiation treatment planning of esophageal cancer: reduction in geographic misses with equal inter-observer variability: PET/CT improves esophageal target definition. Dis Esophagus. 2010;23(6):493–501.
53. Wang YC, Hsieh TC, Yu CY, Yen KY, Chen SW, Yang SN. The clinical application of 4D 18F-FDG PET/CT on gross tumor volume delineation for radiotherapy planning in esophageal squamous cell cancer. J Radiat Res. 2012;53(4):594–600.
54. Muijs CT, Pruim J, Beukema JC, Berveling MJ, Plukker JT, Langendijk JA. Oesophageal tumour progression between the diagnostic 18F-FDG-PET and the 18F-FDG-PET for radiotherapy treatment planning. Radiother Oncol. 2013;106(3):283–7.

Oesophageal and Gastric Malignancy: Pictorial Atlas

10

Anna Paschali and Teresa A. Szyszko

Contents

A. Paschali
Division of Imaging Sciences and Biomedical Engineering, St Thomas' Hospital, Kings
College London, London, UK

T.A. Szyszko (✉)
King's College and Guy's and St Thomas' PET Centre, Division of Imaging Sciences and
Biomedical Engineering, Kings College London, St Thomas' Hospital, London, UK
e-mail: teresa.szyszko-walls@kcl.ac.uk

© Springer International Publishing Switzerland 2016   91
T.A. Szyszko (ed.), *PET/CT in Oesophageal and Gastric Cancer*, Clinicians' Guides
to Radionuclide Hybrid Imaging, DOI 10.1007/978-3-319-29240-3_10

10.1 Case 1: Extensive Primary Oesophageal Tumour with Local and Distant Nodal Disease as Well as Distant Metastases

Clinical Details Seventy-eight-year-old man with newly diagnosed large polypoid poorly differentiated adenocarcinoma of distal oesophagus.

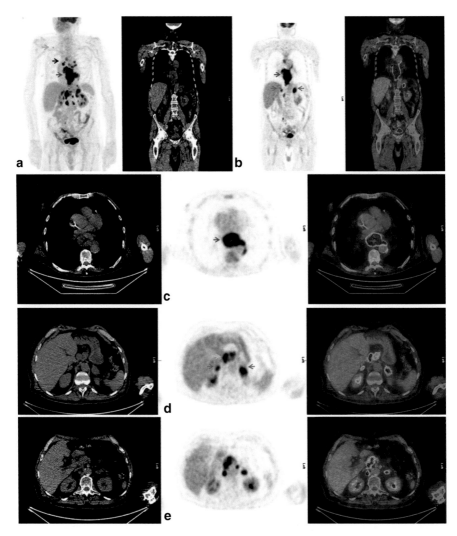

Fig. 10.1 (**a**) Maximum intensity projection (MIP) image; (**b**) coronal images and (**c–e**) axial images of low-dose CT, PET and fused PET-CT. There is high-grade uptake in the primary lesion, which extends from the carina to the distal oesophagus (*red arrow* **a**, **b**). There is circumferential thickening of the oesophageal wall with increased FDG uptake extending out from the primary lesion and wrapping itself around the anterior and lateral descending aorta (*red arrow* **c**). There is involvement of multiple mediastinal lymph nodes (*black arrow* **a**), a small right supraclavicular fossa (SCF) lymph node (*green arrow* **a**), and multiple infradiaphragmatic (coeliac axis and retroperitoneal) lymph nodes (*yellow arrows* **a**, **d** and **e**). There are metastases in both adrenals (*blue arrows* **b**, **d**)

Teaching Points It is difficult to delineate the depth of invasion of oesophageal cancer using FDG-PET-CT. In this case there is a locally advanced oesophageal tumour with possible invasion of the descending aorta and endoscopic ultrasound (EUS) is required for clarification.

Extensive regional and distant nodal involvement is identified, including a small right SCF lymph node which was not identified on the CT scan alone.

Bilateral metabolically active adrenal metastases are visualized. FDG-PET-CT is most useful in detecting distant metastatic disease.

10.2 Case 2: PET-CT and PET-MR Imaging of Extensive Oesophageal Primary Tumour but No Evidence of Nodal or Distant Metastatic Disease

Clinical Details Eighty-year-old patient with an oesophageal stricture. Biopsy revealed adenocarcinoma; CT shows large hiatus hernia and oesophageal thickening.

Teaching Point Even when there is an extensive metabolically active oesophageal primary malignancy, they may not be any evidence of local invasion, nodal disease or metastatic disease.

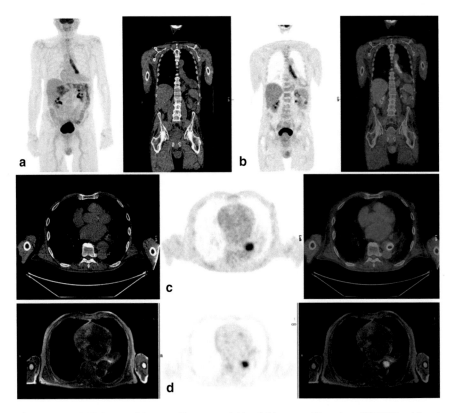

Fig. 10.2 (**a**) MIP image; (**b**) coronal images and (**c**) axial images of low-dose CT, PET and fused PET-CT. There is high-grade uptake in the primary lesion (SUV max = 16.6) involving an extensive length of the mid to distal oesophagus, over a craniocaudal distance of approximately 11 cm, starting just below the carina down to the gastric cardia. No pathologically enlarged or metabolically active regional lymph nodes are demonstrated. (**d**) Axial images of MR (T1 sequence), PET and fused PET-MR of the same patient demonstrating the oesophageal tumour with no evidence of invasion of adjacent structures. In both studies (PET-CT and PET-MR), there is no evidence of nodal involvement or distant metastasis

10.3   Case 3: Primary Oesophageal Tumour with Locoregional Nodal Involvement

Clinical Details   Sixty-seven-year-old patient with squamous cell carcinoma of the oesophagus and a 3 mm hypodense liver lesion.

Teaching Points   Lymph nodes from the cervical region down to and including the coeliac axis are considered to be locoregional nodes and it is the number of nodes that determines the N stage (N1, 1–2; N2, 3–6; and N3 > 7). In this case, the left gastric lymph node is involved. Nodal disease in the direct vicinity of the primary lesion is difficult to detect as uptake in the tumour may obscure peritumoural nodes, resulting in a false-negative study. EUS is the modality of choice in assessing peritumoural nodes. False positives are unusual but could be due to an inflammatory/granulomatous process.

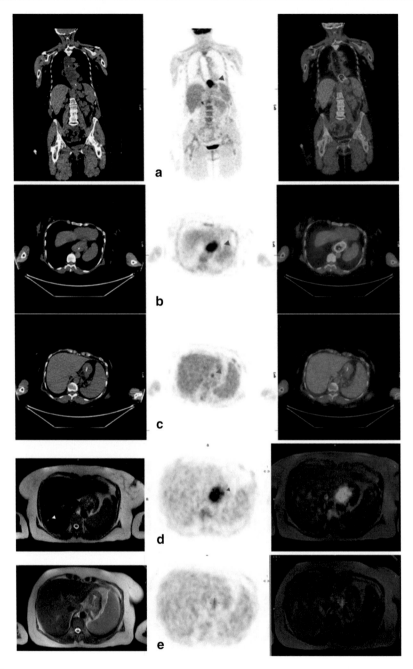

Fig. 10.3 (**a**) Coronal and (**b** and **c**) axial images of low-dose CT, PET and fused PET-CT. (**d**, **e**) Axial images of MR (T2 sequence), PET and fused PET-MR of the same patient. There is high-grade uptake (SUVmax = 11.5) within the lower oesophageal/GOJ tumour (*red arrow* on **a**, **b** and **d** images) and possibly within small paraoesophageal lymph nodes. There is proximal dilatation of the oesophagus and nasogastric tube in situ (**a**). There is a focus of increased FDG uptake in a left gastric region corresponding to a small lymph node (*blue arrow* on **c**, PET marker and *blue arrow* on MRI – **e**). FDG tracer distribution in the liver is within normal limits. On the T2 MR image, a 3 mm cyst or haemangioma is visualized on segment 7 of the liver (*white arrow* **d**)

10.4   Case 4: Oesophageal Tumour with Low-Grade Metabolic Activity

Clinical Details Sixty-five-year-old patient with adenocarcinoma of oesophagus. CT shows lesion extending to the diaphragm and small gastric nodes.

Teaching Point The primary oesophageal tumour demonstrates only low to moderate grade of metabolic activity. Oesophageal tumours, even those which are locally advanced, may show a limited or absent FDG accumulation in well-differentiated tumours (with low GLUT 1 expression) as well as mucus-secreting tumours and/or signet ring cell containing subtypes. When the primary tumour has only low-grade uptake, the sensitivity of PET for the detection of metastases is reduced.

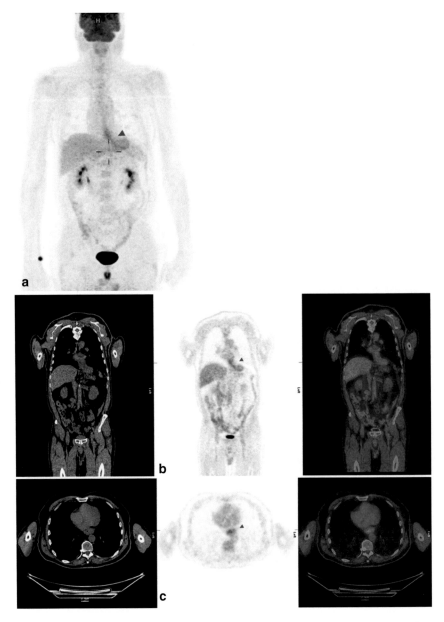

Fig. 10.4 (**a**) MIP; (**b**) coronal images; (**c, d, f** and **g**) axial images of low-dose CT, PET and fused PET-CT, as well as (**e**) axial images of MR (T2), PET and fused PET-MR of the same patient. There is low-grade increased FDG uptake (SUVmax = 4) in the primary lesion in the distal oesophagus extending to the GOJ (*red arrow* **a–c**) with corresponding concentric mural thickening on axial CT images (**c**). Small left gastric nodes are seen in the CT and MR measuring up to 1 cm (*yellow arrow* on **d, e**) which are non-FDG avid. Low-grade tracer uptake is noted in small mediastinal lymph nodes (bilateral paratracheal, *blue arrows* on **f,** and anterior mediastinal, *green arrow* on **g**)

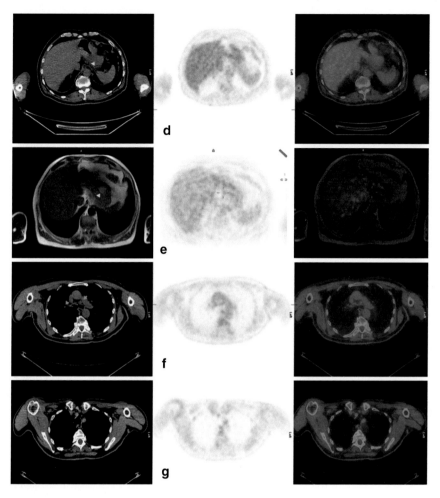

Fig. 10.4 (continued)

10.5   Case 5: Small Primary Oesophageal Tumour with Incidental Uptake in the Sigmoid Colon

Clinical Details Seventy-one-year-old patient with a history of Barrett's oesophagus and a recent diagnosis of high-grade dysplasia/intramucosal adenocarcinoma.

Teaching Points There is low-grade metabolic activity within the known dysplasia/intramucosal adenocarcinoma of the distal oesophagus with no underlying mural abnormality. PET has reduced sensitivity in detecting tumours below its spatial resolution, which is approximately 4–6 mm. Small tumour size is a common cause for false-negative F-18 FDG-PET findings.

In this case PEt also detected a metabolically active lesion in the sigmoid colon and further investigation with colonoscopy was recommended to exclude the possibility of a synchronous second incidental malignancy.

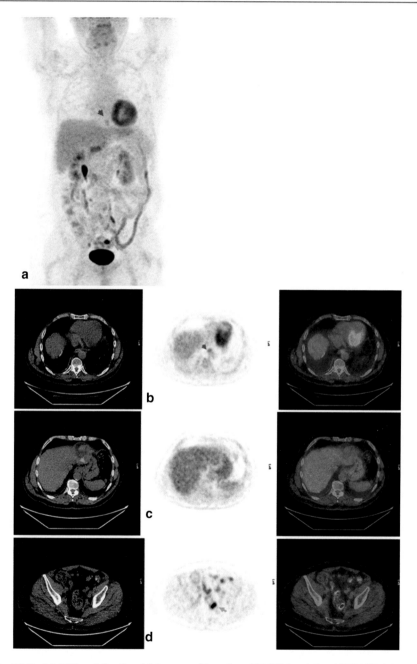

Fig. 10.5 (**a**) MIP and (**b–d**) axial images of low-dose CT, PET and fused PET-CT. There is low-grade FDG uptake in the primary lesion within the distal oesophagus approximately 2 cm from the gastro-oesophageal junction with no apparent mural abnormalities on the CT (SUVmax = 3.7) (*red arrow* **a**, **b**). There is no perceptible uptake within morphologically normal left gastric lymph nodes (*blue arrow* on CT, **c**). In the sigmoid colon there is a discrete focus of intensely increased tracer uptake corresponding to a moderately thickening of the wall (*green arrow* **a**, **d**). This finding is highly suspicious for a synchronous second incidental malignancy

10.6   Case 6: Oesophageal Cancer with Widespread Metastases

Clinical Details Seventy-four-year-old man with lower oesophageal thickening, suspicious nodes, lung nodules and liver abnormalities.

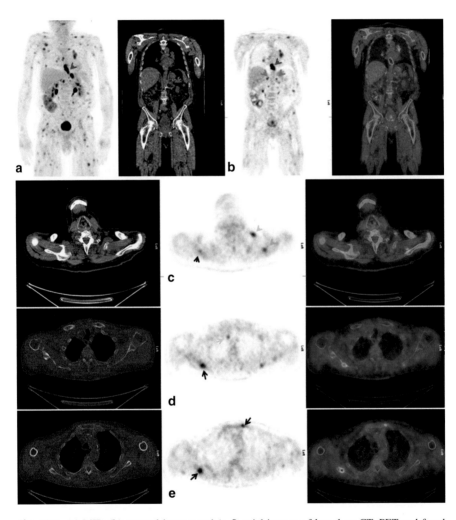

Fig. 10.6 (**a**) MIP; (**b**) coronal images and (**c–f**) axial images of low-dose CT, PET and fused PET-CT. There is a metabolically active lower oesophageal tumour with widespread FDG-avid metastases. In particular there is intense FDG activity associated with thickening of the lower oesophagus down to the gastro-oesophageal junction (*red arrow*) and the proximal stomach. There are numerous metastases involving lymph nodes above and below the diaphragm (*yellow arrows* **c**, **d**), both adrenal glands (*blue arrows* **b**), the skeleton (*black arrows* **c–e**), soft tissues (*green arrows* **f**) and the lungs. Tracer distribution in the liver is unremarkable

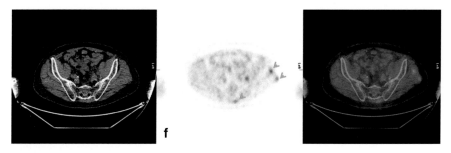

Fig. 10.6 (continued)

Teaching Point   The PET-CT scan showed widespread metastatic disease in lymph nodes, adrenals, skeleton, lungs and muscles. PET imaging reveals more metastatic sites than the CT especially in soft tissues and bones. Distant metastases are present in 20–30 % of oesophageal tumours at initial staging.

10.7   Case 7: Oesophageal Cancer with Locoregional (N) and Distant Nodal (M) Disease

Clinical Details Seventy-two-year-old man with a large mid-oesophageal poorly differentiated/signet ring adenocarcinoma. CT shows bulky primary and nodes below the diaphragm.

Teaching Point Appearances are in keeping with the known oesophageal malignancy with multiple sites of nodal involvement both above and below the diaphragm. The coeliac axis node is in keeping with locoregional nodal (N-stage) involvement, but the left para-aortic nodal disease is in keeping with M1 disease. The right subpleural focal uptake is also likely to represent a further metastatic deposit.

Fig. 10.7 (**a**) MIP image demonstrating the high-grade metabolically active oesophageal malignancy in the distal oesophagus extending through the gastro-oesophageal junction into the gastric cardia. (**b–f**) Axial images of low-dose CT, PET and fused PET-CT demonstrating a metabolically active high paraoesophageal lymph node (**b** *blue arrow*), tumour uptake (**c** *red arrow*), a subpleural focus in the right lower lobe of the lung (**d**, *black arrow*), multiple upper abdominal/coeliac axis nodes (**e**) and a left para-aortic lymph node (**f**)

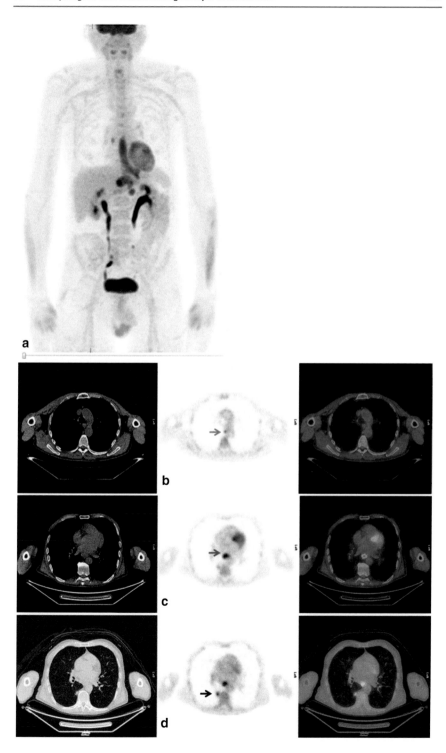

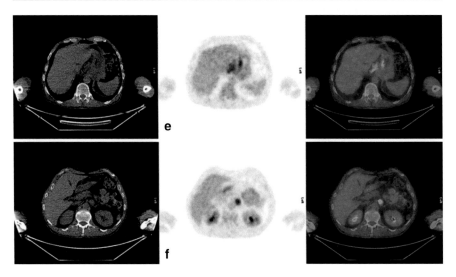

Fig. 10.7 (continued)

10.8   Case 8: Oesophageal Cancer with Extensive Nodal Disease and Vocal Cord Palsy

Clinical Details Seventy-three-year-old man with newly diagnosed ulcerated tumour at GOJ. Biopsy shows intramucosal adenocarcinoma arising in Barrett's oesophagus.

Teaching Points In vocal cord palsy, there are increased physiological uptake in the "normal" cord and absent uptake in the involved cord.

Supraclavicular nodes are considered locoregional (N stage).

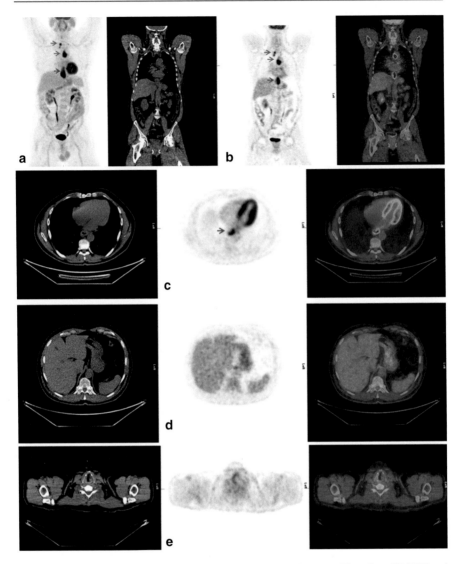

Fig. 10.8 (**a**) MIP image; (**b**) and (**c–e**) coronal images. Axial images of low-dose CT, PET and fused PET-CT. There is intensely increased tracer uptake (SUV max = 16.9) within a 6.8 cm long oesophageal tumour extending from the level of the left atrium to the gastro-oesophageal junction (*red arrow* **a–c**). There are metabolically active small paraoesophageal lymph nodes, as well as bulky aortopulmonary window (*blue arrow* **a**, **b**) and right paratracheal nodes (*blue arrow*, **a**, **b**) and a small left supraclavicular fossa lymph node (*yellow arrow* **a**). There are also a few metabolically active small left gastric/coeliac axis lymph nodes in the upper abdomen (*green arrow* **d**). Note is made of absent uptake in the left vocal cord indicating left vocal cord palsy caused by the bulky aortopulmonary window nodal disease (**e**)

10.9   Case 9: Upstaging Disease by Detecting Distant Bony Metastases

Brief Clinical Details   Seventy-two-year-old female patient with dysphagia. OGD shows high-grade dysplasia (HGD) with transformation to adenocarcinoma. CT shows mural thickening.

Teaching Point   PET-CT has upstaged the patient from T3N0M0 to T3N0M1 by detecting distant bony metastatic disease, not identified on CT, thereby rendering him inoperable. Use of PET-CT helps prevent inappropriate interventions.

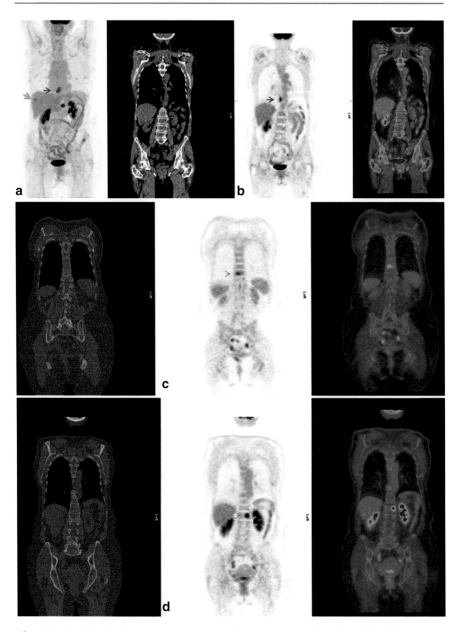

Fig. 10.9 (**a**) MIP; (**b–d**) coronal images and (**e, f**) axial images of low-dose CT, PET and fused PET-CT. There is increased tracer uptake in a segment of mural thickening in the lower oesophagus at the level of T10/T11 (SUV max of 6.7) (*red arrow* **a, b**). There is mild dilatation of the oesophagus proximally. There is no significant uptake in low small volume mediastinal lymph nodes. However there is increased uptake in several foci in the skeleton, specifically in the T10, L1, L3 vertebrae and the anterior aspect of the left iliac crest (*blue arrows* **c–f**) with a corresponding lytic area at the left iliac crest (**f**), while at the other skeletal sites, there is no underlying CT abnormality noted. In the liver there is a focus of increased uptake in the anterior aspect of segment 8 with no underlying abnormality (*green arrow* **a**). Elsewhere tracer distribution is within normal limits

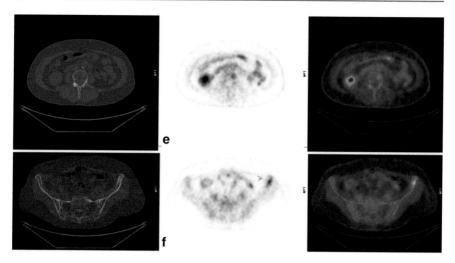

Fig. 10.9 (continued)

10.10 Case 10: Unknown Liver Metastases in Addition to Extensive Nodal Disease

Clinical Details Eighty-seven-year-old man with newly diagnosed adenocarcinoma at the GOJ. CT shows large hiatus hernia as well as aortocaval and paraoesophageal lymph nodes.

Teaching Point The PET scan detected additional metastatic disease in the liver in a patient with known extensive lymphadenopathy. Periportal and retroperitoneal nodes are considered to be M1 stage.

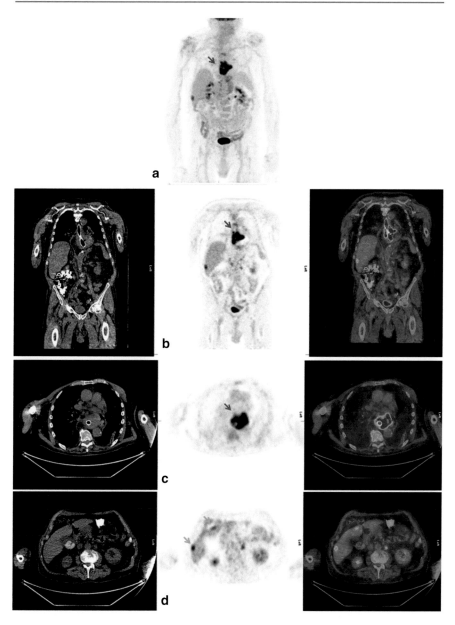

Fig. 10.10 (**a**) MIP; (**b**) coronal images and (**c**, **d**) axial images of low-dose CT, PET and fused PET-CT. The large distal oesophageal/gastro-oesophageal junction tumour demonstrates intensely increased tracer uptake (SUV max = 14.9) (*red arrow* **a–c**). There is involvement of several lymph nodes above and below the diaphragm, including paraoesophageal, subcarinal, paratracheal, right paracardiac, retrocrural, portal, aortocaval and left para-aortic lymph nodes (**c**, **d**). Two foci of intense tracer uptake are noted in segment 6 and segment 5/4b of the liver (*green arrows* **d**)

10.11 Case 11: Locally Invasive Oesophageal Malignancy with Tracheo-Oesophageal Fistula Formation

Clinical Details Seventy-three-year-old man with newly diagnosed moderately differentiated squamous cell carcinoma. CT shows proximal oesophageal thickening and a trachea-oesophageal fistula as well as nonspecific mediastinal lymph nodes and a right lung lesion.

PMH: hemi-hepatectomy for HCC 2013.

Teaching Points The mediastinal lymph nodes, particularly the right paratracheal/precarinal node, appear suspicious for malignancy and biopsy is advised prior to further treatment. Mediastinal nodes are considered to be N stage.

The cavitating nodule in the right upper lobe appears to be inflammatory/infective in nature and uptake in the hilar nodes may simply be reactive.

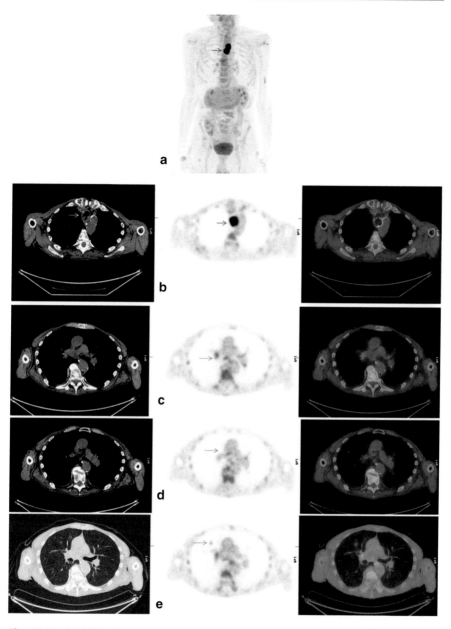

Fig. 10.11 (**a**) MIP; (**b–e**) axial images of low-dose CT, PET and fused PET-CT. The mid-oesophageal tumour shows high-grade tracer uptake (SUVmax=20.6) (*red arrows* **a**, **b**) and indents into the posterior trachea, where there is a fistula (*white arrow* **b**). There is moderately increased tracer uptake within enlarged right lower paratracheal/precarinal lymph node, bilateral hilar nodes and a smaller subcarinal lymph node (*blue arrows* **c**, **d**). A cavitating nodule is visualized in the right upper lobe of the lung with low-grade tracer uptake (*green arrow* **e**). There is moderately diffusely increased bone marrow uptake (likely reactive). Elsewhere bone review reveals an osteophyte at T7 and a small focus of sclerosis in the right iliac bone with no associated FDG uptake

10.12 Case 12: Bony Metastases with Suspicion of Invasion into Spinal Canal

Clinical Details Seventy-seven-year-old man with an upper oesophageal mass, suspicious for malignancy a right lung nodule – ? a pulmonary metastasis.

Teaching Point When there is suspicion of invasion into the spinal canal, an urgent MRI is required to assess for spinal cord compromise.

Fig. 10.12 (**a**) MIP; (**b–h**) axial images of low-dose CT, PET and fused PET-CT; (**f, g**) sagittal fused images. There is a metabolically active oesophageal malignancy with perioesophageal nodes (*red arrow* **a, b**) and direct invasion of the T1, T3 and T4 vertebrae causing osseous destruction. In particular there are a lytic area in the body of T1 (*arrow* **d, f**), severe destruction of the T3 vertebra with lysis (*yellow arrow* **e, f**) and a suspicion of extension into the spinal canal. Another skeletal focus is visualized in the posterior left aspect of the T11 vertebral body with no underlying lysis on the CT (*white arrow* **g**). Two confluent nodal masses with necrotic centres are seen in the right supraclavicular fossa and a small node in the left supraclavicular fossa (*green arrows* **a, c**). A 10 mm nodule is noted in the low lower lobe of the lung with low-grade uptake (*arrow*, **h**). The left lower lobe lung nodule probably also represents a metastasis, but could conceivably be inflammatory given its low-grade uptake

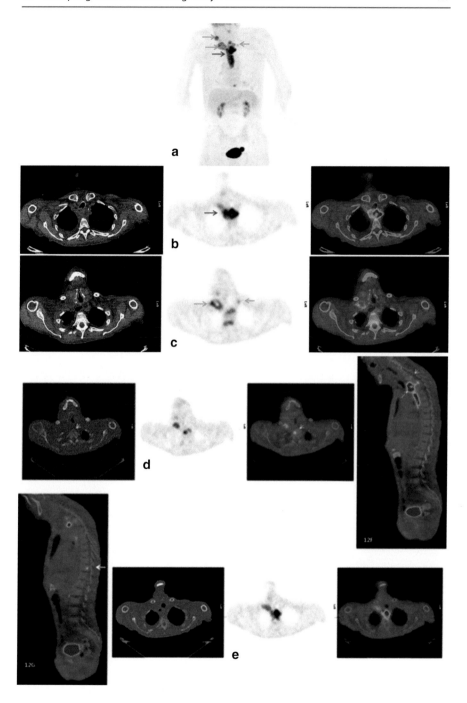

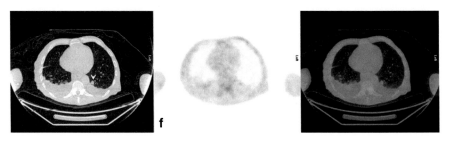

Fig. 10.12 (continued)

10.13 Case 13: Neck Nodes with Histologically Proven Squamous Cell Carcinoma But Unknown Primary

Clinical Details Seventy-year-old lady with enlarged left lower neck nodes. Biopsy of a level 4 cervical lymph node showed squamous cell carcinoma (SCC). Where is the primary?

Teaching Points Squamous cell carcinoma in cervical nodes is most commonly due to a primary malignancy within the head and neck. In this case, the unknown primary lesion was within the oesophagus. Distant nodal metastases, beyond the coeliac axis, are classed as M1 disease.

In the upper two-thirds of the oesophagus, squamous cell carcinomas (SCCs) predominate, with alcohol and smoking being the main risk factors. Carcinomas of the distal oesophagus/gastro-oesophageal junction, on the other hand, are mostly adenocarcinomas.

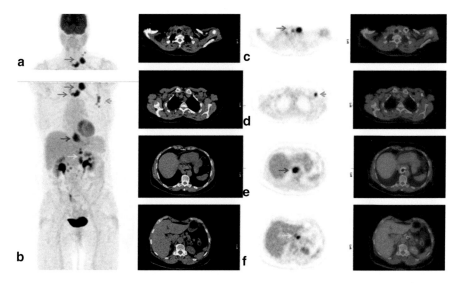

Fig. 10.13 MIP images of the head and neck (**a**) and half body (**b**). (**c–f**) Axial images of low-dose CT, PET and fused PET-CT. There are multiple metabolically active left cervical nodes from levels III–V extending to the superior mediastinum (*blue arrows* **a–c**). Increased tracer uptake is also noted in the left axillary lymph nodes (*green arrow* **d**). There is a 4 cm segment of the distal oesophagus extending to the gastro-oesophageal junction with mural thickening and intensely increased tracer uptake (SUVmax = 10.0) (*red arrow*). Further increased uptake of tracer is noted in several left gastric, coeliac, superior mesenteric, para-aortic, aortocaval and paracaval lymph nodes (e.g. *yellow arrow*, **f**). The FDG distribution elsewhere and in particular the head and neck region is physiological

10.14 Case 14: Treatment Response

Clinical Details Sixty-six-year-old man with moderately differentiated adenocarcinoma of the lower oesophagus. T3N3M1 at baseline scan with a solitary metastasis on femur. Completed six cycles primary chemotherapy. Response to treatment assessment.

Teaching Point FDG-PET is useful for evaluating the response to chemotherapy as, in contrast to CT or MRI, it can distinguish viable tumour tissue from fibrotic or necrotic tissue.

Fig. 10.14 MIP and several axial fused PET-CT images (**a–e**) of the same patient at the baseline and post-treatment assessment demonstrating complete metabolic response to treatment with a considerable decrease in size and metabolic activity with only minor distal oesophageal thickening on the low-dose CT, complete resolution of the mediastinal lymphadenopathy and the right femur skeletal site and only low-grade uptake associated with a small left gastric lymph node (*white arrow* **d**, post-treatment)

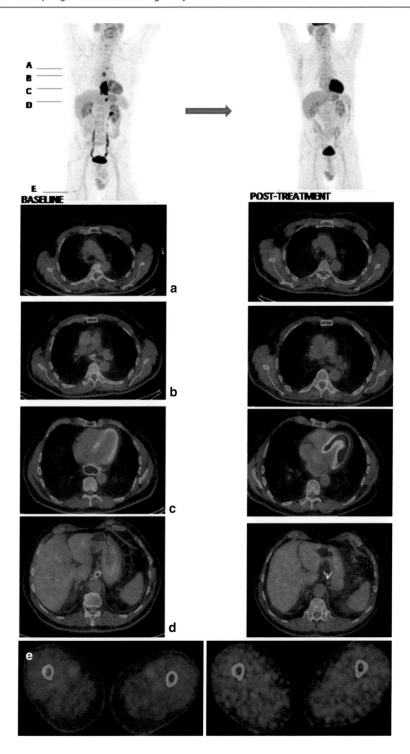

10.15 Case 15: Treatment Response

Clinical Details Fourty-seven-year-old lady with a lower oesophageal cancer. Initial staging: T3N2M0. Completed primary chemotherapy. Chest infection (with CXR changes at left base). Evaluation of response to treatment.

Teaching Point Partial metabolic response to treatment with residual activity only within the primary tumour in the gastro-oesophageal junction but resolution of disease elsewhere, potentially altering the management plan. FDG decrease after therapy has been shown to correlate closely to histopathological outcome. Persistent FDG uptake post treatment has been shown to correlate with residual tumour and poor survival.

Fig. 10.15 MIP and several axial images of low-dose CT, PET and fused PET-CT at baseline and post-treatment. There has been a significant reduction in the size and the metabolic activity associated with the gastro-oesophageal tumour. There is a residual activity within the primary tumour in the gastro-oesophageal junction (*yellow arrow*). Uptake previously identified in portal, peripancreatic and left gastric nodes has resolved

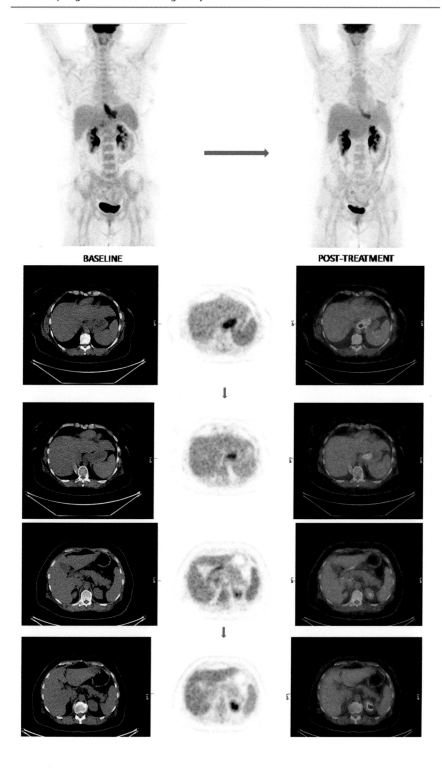

10.16 Case 16: Treatment Response

Clinical Details Seventy-one-year-old man with squamous cell carcinoma of the mid-oesophagus including a supraclavicular fossa (SCF) lymph node positive on baseline PET. Completed three cycles of chemotherapy. Treatment response assessment.

Teaching Point New foci of uptake within the lung post chemotherapy most likely have an inflammatory/infective aetiology but should be followed up.

If a patient receives radiotherapy, post-radiotherapy oesophagitis can demonstrate significant uptake for 12 weeks and hence it is best to rescan after this time has elapsed. Similarly, post-operative inflammation persists for 4–6 weeks and hence it is best to wait for at least 6 weeks before re-scanning the patient.

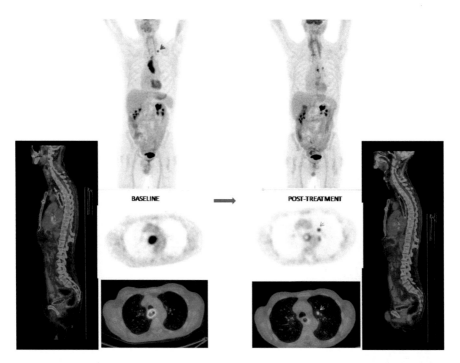

Fig. 10.16 MIP, axial and sagittal images at baseline post-treatment PET-CT assessment. There is uptake in a 10 mm left supraclavicular lymph node at baseline (*red arrow* on MIP). After treatment, there has been complete resolution of uptake at this site. There has also been a significant reduction of the metabolic activity at the site of the original primary and the degree of oesophageal wall thickening has also significantly reduced. The oesophagus has been stented and there is increased uptake, likely inflammatory, at the inferior and superior aspects of the stent. There are several foci of high-grade tracer uptake scattered throughout the left upper lobe on the post-treatment scan (e.g. *arrow* on axial post-treatment image), corresponding to areas of ill-defined nodular consolidation

10.17   Case 17: Surveillance Imaging

Clinical Details   Sixty-nine-year-old man with T3N1M0 adenocarcinoma of the oesophagus cancer underwent neoadjuvant chemotherapy, thoracoabdominal oesophagectomy and adjuvant chemotherapy. Surveillance CT 1 year later shows bulky anastomosis and new adrenal lesion.

Teaching Point   FDG-PET is an extremely useful modality for detecting not only locoregional recurrence but also distant metastatic recurrence.

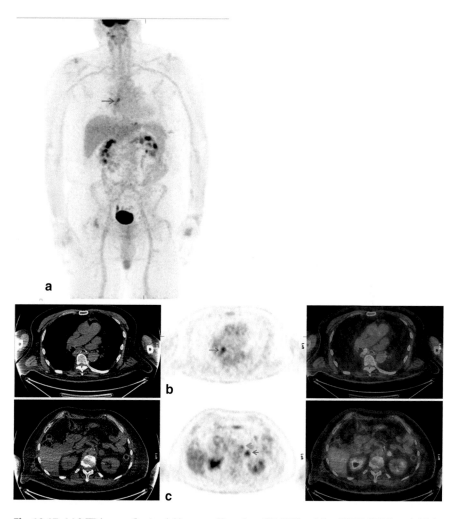

Fig. 10.17 (**a**) MIP image; (**b**, **c**) axial images of low-dose CT, PET and fused PET-CT. There is high-grade increased tracer uptake associated with the thickening in the gastro-oesophageal anastomosis (*red arrow* **a**, **b**). There is high-grade uptake in a left adrenal mass (*blue arrow* **c**). There is also a small, moderately avid lymph node just to the left of the SMA trunk (*green arrow* **c**). Appearances are suggestive of recurrence at the anastomosis with a new left adrenal metastasis and an upper abdominal node

10.18 Case 18: Surveillance Imaging

Clinical Details Seventy-one-year-old lady with previous locally advanced moderate to poorly differentiated adenocarcinoma of the oesophagus (T2N0M0) who underwent transhiatal oesophagectomy and chemotherapy. Three years later there is a new soft tissue mass in oesophagus identified on CT. Is this recurrence?

Teaching Point A typical case of tumour recurrence within the gastric pull-up.

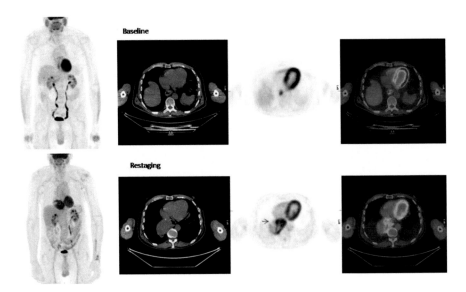

Fig. 10.18 MIP and axial images of low-dose CT, PET and fused PET-CT at baseline and restaging scan. In the restaging scan there is a large area of heterogeneously increased FDG uptake (SUVmax = 11.6) within the gastric pull-up indicating recurrent disease (*red arrow*). There is no evidence of nodal disease or distant metastasis

10.19   Case 19: Signet Ring Cell Gastric Cancer

Clinical Details Fifty-six-year-old lady with newly diagnosed poorly differentiated adenocarcinoma with signet ring cells on the greater curve of the stomach. CT
shows distal stomach primary with mesenteric nodularity of unknown
significance.

The focal area of moderate uptake within the lesser curve of the stomach may relate
to tumour with adjacent inflammation or possibly the biopsy site.

Teaching Point FDG uptake in signet ring cell carcinoma is low due to the low
GLUT-1 expression. In these cases the sensitivity of PET for the detection of metastases is reduced.

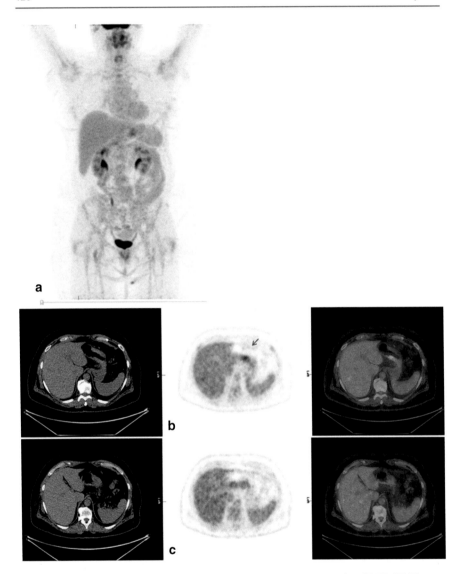

Fig. 10.19 (**a**) MIP image; (**b**, **c**) axial images of low-dose CT, PET and fused PET-CT. The area of thickening within the distal fundus of the stomach demonstrates only very low-grade/background FDG uptake over the majority of its extent (**a**, *blue arrow*); however there is a small area of moderately increased uptake along the inferior lesser curve (**a**, *yellow arrow*). The area of mesenteric nodularity and stranding (**c**) demonstrates only low-grade FDG uptake. No enlarged or metabolically active local regional lymph nodes are identified

10.20 Case 20: Gastric Adenocarcinoma

Clinical Details Sixty-five-year-old man with poorly differentiated adenocarcinoma, large mobile lesser curve tumour 5 cm and left gastric LNs at laparoscopy, CT T4 N2 ?M1, lesser curve thickening with nodes at the porta hepatis and in the left gastric region.

Findings are consistent with gastric carcinoma and involved left gastric lymph nodes. Uptake related to anterior abdominal wall could relate to recent laparoscopy and uptake at a port site, but it is very intense and clinical correlation is advised to exclude a soft tissue metastasis/Sister Mary Joseph nodule.

Teaching Point The Sister Mary Joseph nodule is a palpable nodule bulging into the umbilicus as a result of metastasis of a malignant cancer in the pelvis or abdomen. Gastrointestinal malignancies account for about half of these (most commonly gastric cancer, colonic cancer or pancreatic cancer).

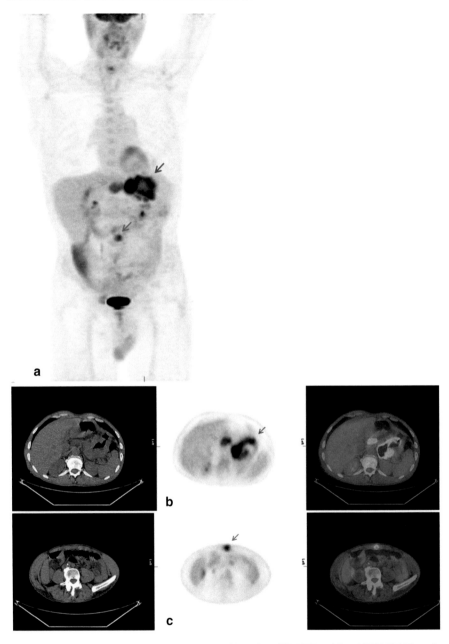

Fig. 10.20 (**a**) MIP image; (**b**, **c**) axial images of low-dose CT, PET and fused PET-CT. There is intensely increased tracer uptake (SUV max = 7.1) within the large gastric tumour centred on the lesser curve of the stomach (**a**, **b**, *red arrow*). There are FDG-avid left gastric nodes (**a**, **b** *green arrow*). In the midline anterior abdominal wall, there is a focus of high uptake (**a**, **c** *blue arrow*) corresponding to soft tissue thickening on the CT component

Appendix 1: Regional Lymph Node Stations for Staging Esophageal Cancer

Locoregional (N stage) disease was redefined in the seventh edition of the AJCC Cancer Staging Manual as any periesophageal lymph node from cervical nodes to celiac nodes and subclassified by the number of involved nodes (N0 = 0; N1 = 1 − 2; N2 = 3 − 6; N4 > 7).

Supraclavicular and mediastinal nodes are considered N stage.

Metastatic (M stage) disease is simply M1 or M0 (and the subclassifications M1a, M1b, and Mx, used in the sixth edition, have been removed). Periportal and retroperitoneal nodes are considered M1.

© Springer International Publishing Switzerland 2016
T.A. Szyszko (ed.), *PET/CT in Oesophageal and Gastric Cancer,* Clinicians' Guides
to Radionuclide Hybrid Imaging, DOI 10.1007/978-3-319-29240-3

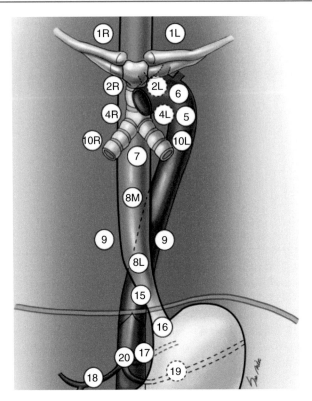

Courtesy of Hong SJ, et al. New TNM staging system for esophageal cancer: what chest radiologists need to know. Radiographics. 2014;34(6):1722–40. Regional lymph nodes according to the seventh edition of the staging manual for esophageal cancer. 1L left supraclavicular, 1R right supraclavicular, 2L left upper paratracheal, 2R right upper paratracheal, 4L left lower paratracheal, 4R right lower paratracheal, 5 aortopulmonary, 6 nterior mediastinal, 7 subcarinal, 8L lower paraesophageal, 8M middle paraesophageal, 9 pulmonary ligament, 10L left tracheobronchial, 10R right tracheobronchial, 15 diaphragmatic, 16 aracardial, 17 left gastric, 18 common hepatic, 19 splenic, 20 celiac. The posterior mediastinal lymph node (3P) is not shown

Index

© Springer International Publishing Switzerland 2016
T.A. Szyszko (ed.), *PET/CT in Oesophageal and Gastric Cancer*, Clinicians' Guides to Radionuclide Hybrid Imaging, DOI 10.1007/978-3-319-29240-3

Printed in the United States
By Bookmasters